the dramatic life *of a* country doctor

fifty years of disasters and diagnoses

Dr. Arnold Burden

with Andrew Safer

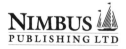

NIMBUS PUBLISHING LTD

This book is dedicated to my wife, Helen, who has been with me most of these fifty years, and to my children, Bill, Kent, David, and Tim.

Nimbus Publishing Limited
3731 Mackintosh St, Halifax, NS B3K 5A5
(902) 455-4286 nimbus.ca

Printed and bound in Canada

Design: Jenn Embree

Library and Archives Canada Cataloguing in Publication

Burden, Arnold, 1922-
The dramatic life of a country doctor : fifty years of
disasters and diagnoses / Arnold Burden ; with Andrew
Safer. — Updated ed.
Previous title: Fifty years of emergencies (original ISBN 0-88999-500-1)
ISBN 978-1-55109-872-2

1. Burden, Arnold, 1922-. 2. Physicians—Nova Scotia—Biography.
I. Safer, Andrew II. Title.

R464.B897A3 2011   610.92   C2011-903913-3

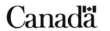 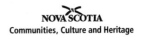

Nimbus Publishing acknowledges the financial support for its publishing activities from the Government of Canada through the Canada Book Fund (CBF) and the Canada Council for the Arts, and from the Province of Nova Scotia through the Department of Communities, Culture and Heritage.

Contents

Preface   1

1. The Bay Ice Story   3

2. The Dirty Thirties   7

3. A Close Call at Sea   21

4. Heavy Casualties   37

5. Sandbostel Concentration Camp   53

6. Veteran, Student, Miner, and Doctor   69

7. Reviving a Dead Man and the Interminable Maternity   87

8. Surgery on a Horsehair Sofa, A Mysterious Suicide, and Murder by Mistake   107

9. The Mine Explosion: Rescuing the Trapped Men   119

10. The Fire that Gobbled Up Main Street   135

11. The Bump: Burial or Nightmare   141

12. More Rescues and the *Ed Sullivan Show*   159

13. Wringing Urine from Diapers and Other Rewards   175

Preface

MY CAREER BEGAN UNINTENTIONALLY WHEN I PERFORMED MY FIRST SURGERY IN THE WOODS, AND THE SHOCK OF WORLD WAR Two then catapulted me into my next training ground: No. 7 Canadian General Hospital in England. As a medical orderly and then a hospital clerk, I handled bombing casualties and then battle casualties after D-Day in France, Belgium, Holland, and Germany.

After medical school in Halifax, Nova Scotia, I took over a country practice in Prince Edward Island where I learned the kind of medical care that's not taught in books. Back home in Springhill, Nova Scotia, I was the first doctor to enter the mines after the No. 4 Mine Explosion and the No. 2 Mine Bump, and worked along with the underground rescue teams to bring the gassed and trapped miners to the surface. Later, each rescuer was honoured to receive the ribbon of the Carnegie Hero Award. After the disasters I have kept up both hospital and office practices, and became medical officer for a 450-man prison.

From removing a shotgun pellet from the leg of a friend using a hunting knife at age fourteen to performing surgery in a farm kitchen, elevating a man's skull bone that had pressed into the brain tissue, I have never known what's around the corner.

During my country practice, in the wintertime it was commonplace to make house calls in a car or by horse and sleigh over "winter roads"—that is, through orchards, across fields, and alongside the woods, leaving the snowplows far behind. One spring, after seeing a farm tractor sink three feet into the soft mud, I had to drive 150 miles through back roads to treat a child suffering a 106 degree-fever—my longest house call.

Standing on the draw bar of a tractor or on an open railway trolley car to get past the snow or mud is not the ordinary means of travel for most doctors. Nor is travelling over bay ice in a car with the front doors roped open, while a truck with ladders follows behind in case the car breaks through.

Surgery in an operating room is not the same as being asked to amputate a leg a mile underground in a mine disaster. Discovering that a lobster trap head makes a dandy holder for an IV fluid bottle was one of the many surprises that came from working in rural areas, where resourcefulness was king.

When my own son was critically ill, my wife and I sat at his emergency room bedside day and night. This was when I had my first painfully personal glimpse of the life and death nature of my work.

As a child I had medical coverage under the first pre-paid medical plan in Canada, a check-off at the Springhill mine. Later I paid the check-off when I worked in the mines during summer vacations and then the tables were turned when I became a doctor and was paid the check-off.

I have been honoured to become a senior member of both the Canadian Medical Society and the Nova Scotia Medical Society, but to me the real satisfaction in life has come from helping people. And I've had my share of opportunities these fifty years.

1. *The Bay Ice Story*

Late February, 1954
St. Peter's Bay, Prince Edward Island

I AM STIRRING THE MILK INTO MY MORNING TEA AS I STAND BEFORE THE BIG BAY WINDOW IN THE LIVING ROOM. FROST HAS crept into the corners of the smallish panes. The sun is brilliant. Yesterday's blizzard is a fleeting thought. The screeching forlorn cry of an occasional gull violates the quiet. Not a sprig of greenery is in sight; everything is white, except for the reckless slate grey rocks that push through the snow at the water's edge. They seem to stab at the sky in triumph.

High winds have randomly denuded the icy surface of the bay. Blue-green patches stand out against the mounds, drifts, and pockets of snow. The sunlight picks up rainbows in the ice crystals as they blow across the frozen desert.

"This is good news for my paperwork," pops into my mind.

Maternities, coroner's inquests, and a slew of children's ailments have kept me going until eleven o'clock at night for the past week. "I hope there aren't any emergencies, because I won't be able to get to them." As the last sip of tea sloshes across my tongue, I head for the office just beyond the living room.

A sheet of paper stands at alert in my typewriter. I am hammering out a supply order to Anglo Canadian Drug Company: blood pressure pills, cough syrups, and stomach medicines.

Striking the "n" key, I'm dumbfounded by the sound I least expected: the doorbell.

"How in the hell could anyone get through the drifts on these roads?" I mutter, crossing the hallway. "Must be a neighbour...."

A husky man is standing out front. His face is barely visible beneath a hooded wool coat and the thick grey scarf he's stretched tightly across his face. He yanks on it to speak and I recognize Ian McNeil from across the bay.

"You can say no if you wish, and I wouldn't blame you," he begins haltingly. "But my wife is bleeding badly...." His eyes search mine and hope overcomes timidity. The fact that I'm the only doctor for twenty miles has something to do with it. Finally, he blurts out: "Could you come?"

"How did you possibly get here?" I ask, measuring each word.

"We crossed the ice in a car."

"Well, if you're crazy enough to do that, I'm crazy enough to go back with you." I grab my medical case and load it up with intravenous fluids, IV tubing, syringes, needles, plasma expanders[1], and pitocin.[2] I climb into my down-filled flight suit, pull down the ear-lugs on my Russian hat, lace up my heavy fur-lined boots, and slide on my fleece-lined gloves. In the kitchen I tell my wife, "Helen, there's a woman hemorrhaging in Greenwich and I'm going there...across the ice." I step outside.

Snow blinded and wind-whipped, I follow Ian across the buried lawn. The wedge-shaped bay draws to a point at St. Peter's River, about a half mile from the house. Straight across the bay it's just one mile, but it's six miles to Greenwich. As we tromp through the drifts, I'm thinking of the Midgell and Morell rivers. The flowing water melts the ice where they empty into the bay, and then the surface freezes over, making the ice only inches thick. But we won't be able to recognize these deathtraps because of the drifts.

I stop dead on the other side of the railroad tracks. There, at the bay's edge, is a black sedan with its front doors wide open. A heavy sisal rope crosses the windshield and disappears in double knots on the two window frames. "This is not a routine car ride," I remark dryly. Farther out on the ice is a dark blue pickup truck. A twenty-foot aluminum extension ladder is tied to the hood.

"What's that for?" I cry. My host clears his throat. He's probably wondering if I'm turning chicken.

"Can't be too sure about the ice," he says softly.

With a sinking feeling in my stomach I climb onto the passenger seat. I'm thinking that the woman may lose her life if she continues to hemorrhage, and my jaws tighten. Suddenly I recall a French play I read in college: *No Exit*. The title takes on a new meaning.

"We didn't have any problem on the way over," says Ian, a little too enthusiastically. "But we might as well leave the doors open on the way back. You never know."

Our take-off imprints a semi-circle into the ice's edge, and we begin to make our way cautiously across the bay, the pickup trailing us by a good hundred yards. "No good having him too close if we go through" is my not-so-comforting thought as I look back at our potential saviour. Even with the frigid wind raging inside the car, the sound of the ice crackling under the tires is all I notice.

I know Ian is following the same safe path he took on the way over, but my heart's not convinced—it's in my mouth. We do, in fact, miss the weak spots.

Ian pulls up to the shoreline and parks. Shore grasses poke out of snowdrifts on either side of the trail winding up to Ian's farmhouse. His wife, as it turns out, is having a miscarriage and losing lots of blood. I give her medication and put ice packs on her abdomen. This slows down the bleeding and gets her out of danger. Now she's at the mercy of the snowplows; she'll go to hospital as soon as they open the roads.

I charge five dollars for the house call and a dollar for medication. Ian and I fortify ourselves with mugs of hot tea and homemade strawberry jam on white bread, and then we step outside. From a distance the car, with its roped-open doors, looks like a waiting bird of prey. We inch our way onto the bay highway. The faithful pickup bird-dogs us from a distance. This time, entrusting my life to the mercy of frozen water doesn't seem quite so absurd...seven on a scale of one to ten.

Back at the house, we shake hands. Ian doesn't say much; his eyes do. Inside, I tell Helen what happened, peel off my outer clothes, and sit back down at the typewriter. After counting my blessings, I take out the half-finished supply order and insert a fresh piece of paper to write the bay ice story.

NOTES

1. Plasma expander: A fluid that fills up the veins with substitute plasma to prevent the patient from going into shock.

2. Pitocin: A drug that causes the uterus to contract.

2. *The Dirty Thirties*

I GREW UP DURING THE DEPRESSION IN SPRINGHILL, NOVA SCOTIA. THE LIFEBLOOD OF OUR TOWN HAD SLOWED TO A trickle, with the coal mines working only a third of the time. We called it the "Dirty Thirties"—times were tough.

We were poor but we didn't know it, since we were all in the same boat—except when Buddo Walsh, a doctor's son, came to visit his grandparents across the road from me. Little did I know that I myself would become a doctor, after coming home from the war.

By the time I was born in 1922, Springhill had already attracted close to six thousand settlers, compared to less than five thousand today. About two thousand men worked in the five mines: numbers 1, 2, 4, 6, and 7. My grandfather, George W. Burden, had come from Stellarton around the turn of the century, and later became manager of two of the mines.

Each coal mine is like a town, bustling with dozens of occupations. There are carpenters, labourers, stonedusters who throw fine stone dust on the face of the coal to prevent it from catching fire, water pumpers who keep the mine from flooding, trip drivers who run the coal trolleys up and down the mine slopes, trappers who open and slam doors for ventilation and also to let the trolleys in and out, and—finally—the miners, who swing their picks at the coal face.

Mother died when I was four. No one ever told me what it

was from, but I've always figured it was complications of childbirth. My sister, Audrey, is one and a half years younger than me. I have a few scattered memories of Mother, mostly from when she was sick. But one that really sticks in my mind was the time I never even saw her. I stood out in the street in front of Grandma's home, watching her funeral procession.

Dad was a machinist and a lathe operator. He machined parts for locomotives, and for anything that broke down in the mines. Since broken parts had to be fixed before the next shift, he had more work than the average Springhiller. In those days before the war, that meant three days a week instead of one or two.

As kids, we were noisy most of the time, except at 6:00 PM—time for the mine whistle to blow. That was the only time Audrey and I sat still: if we didn't hear a "WHOO" that meant there would be work the next day.

The men earned two to three dollars a day. With two days of work a week, twenty-four dollars a month had to support a family. There were no mortgages since everyone built their own homes, and most families weren't privileged to have upkeep on automobiles. This was way before the days of Employment Insurance and Old Age Security. But we had something that was unique in Canada at that time: a pre-paid medical plan, called a "check-off" at the mines. Twenty-five cents came out of Dad's pay each week to cover the medical needs of our entire family, including doctor's visits, surgery, maternity care, and medications.

Back then we could get by with very little money, unlike today. Nowadays, our refrigerators' compressors show up on our monthly electric bills as a matter of course; we don't even think of the cost. Refrigerators and freezers didn't even exist in Springhill in the Dirty Thirties. Instead, we used "dummy waiters" in the summertime for lowering the milk, butter, and cheese into the basement where the mud walls would keep the perishables cool.

Everybody hunted, fished, and tended their own gardens. When you shot a deer or moose, you had to give most of it away since you couldn't keep meat without a freezer. The women baked, canned, and made preserves, and the kids went berry picking in late June and July on the outskirts of town. Despite hard times, we were never hungry—except that all kids are always hungry. In fact, my neighbour Pleaman and I often ate two suppers, one at his place and one at mine.

As for the flowers that exploded in our backyard gardens, even they came in handy on special occasions. Each year before Decoration Day—the first Sunday after Labour Day—we would cut the cemetery grass and weed the plots. After a service in remembrance of the departed, we would visit our family graves and then lavish them with dahlias, snapdragons, gladioluses, and roses—a far cry from the plastic or silk flowers you see today, or even the ones that are store bought. Our flowers meant more since they came from our own gardens.

"Indoor plumbing" meant we had a cold water pipe running into the house. To get hot water, we diverted the water through a coil in the coal stove, so the stove had to be going. Instead of toilets we had "backhouses," which were open season for pranks on Halloween. The older boys would sneak around and tip them over. I remember the time when a neighbour decided he would catch the culprits, so he craftily hid inside. Somehow the boys caught on to his ruse, so they promptly locked the door from the outside and then tipped over the whole works. Putting aside the poor fellow's misfortune, this turned out to be a costly "trick" because the home radio aerial had been attached to the backhouse. By the time that neighbour managed to fight his way out, the pranksters were long gone. His backhouse ploy had backfired.

There were no televisions yet, but most families had radios. One of my buddies told me how I could make one from the scrap parts of a telephone I found in the junkyard. First, I took lead and sulphur and put them in the red coal ashes of the kitchen stove to make galena crystals. Then, using wire from the old telephone, I formed two different-sized coils and backed each of them with cardboard. By carefully touching a "cat whisker"—a curved piece of wire—to the different sections of the crystal, and holding the coils on either side, I was able to pick up music from the radio signal! I wound up with my own tubeless radio at age twelve. And it didn't cost a nickel.

In the Dirty Thirties, if you wanted something bad enough, you found out how to get it for free—or you went without it. Stealing was simply not done, so we had to be creative. Someone once said, "Necessity is the mother of invention." Perhaps today's children aren't so inventive since everything is handed to them ready-made.

Audrey and I would each get a dime a week when Dad could afford it. Sometimes we would blow our fortunes at the silent movies, and then race back to tell the story and the latest Tarzan serial to our friends who couldn't afford to come along.

Skating was one of our favourite pastimes. For Christmas we could count on getting a new pair of skates if our old ones were worn out or outgrown. We skated on two of the company ponds; we were not allowed on the third one because of the warm water that was continuously being pumped from the mines. Each winter we had a goof-proof way of knowing when the ice was safe enough for skating. After several days of cold weather Eddie Fraser or his sister, who lived near the ponds, would fall through the ice once or twice. After that, we knew the ice was thick enough.

The way I learned how to swim was very effective, but I don't recommend it for everyone. After picking wild raspberries one day, I went down to the brook. The swimming hole was simply a deep hole in the brook. I climbed onto a raft along with my two neighbours, the Pyke brothers. When we were all aboard, it started to tip. The three of us instinctively moved to the opposite side, and, of course, over it went. My comrades were rescued by their older brothers who were looking on from shore, while I was left to sputter and paddle for myself. Somehow, I ended up on dry land. That was the only swimming lesson I ever needed.

By the time I was in high school, I wanted to earn some extra money. We developed a routine. In early summer, my friends and I would pick wild strawberries—which we brought home for pies and preserves—and then we'd go after the raspberries, which we sold to neighbours. In the morning we'd go to Harry Green's horse pasture on the south end of town to pick a quart of berries. After dinner, we'd pick another quart before going for a swim. Those two quarts were worth fifty cents—not bad pocket change in the Dirty Thirties.

Another money-making scheme was to sell clothes poles for the outdoor clotheslines. We would head for the woods with hatchets and each come back with two or three poles of maple or birch—about two inches in diameter and eight feet tall. They were worth fifteen to twenty-five cents apiece. But since the poles lasted for many years and no one told us about planned obsolescence, our business dwindled. New home building didn't keep up with our industriousness.

At the end of grade ten, I took a job as district agent for the Curtis Publishing Company of Philadelphia. The company published three magazines at the time: *The Saturday Evening Post* (which sold for five cents as a weekly), and two monthlies: *The Ladies' Home Journal* and *Country Gentleman*. I earned one cent per copy sold. For this cent first I had to clear customs, and then retrieve the magazines from the freight shed about a mile from my house. With no car, I had to lug them back either on a cart or a sled, depending on the weather. Next I delivered them to the stores, and to the boys who sold them door to door. I made deliveries on a foot-and-a-half-long "scooter skate," which had roller skate wheels, a forerunner of today's skateboards. Finally, I collected the money and remitted it to the company, along with the tops of the front pages of the unsold copies. I kept this job until I left Springhill to attend grade twelve at Cumberland County Academy in Amherst.

The summer before grade twelve, I went to Westbrook, about twenty miles west of Springhill, to pick strawberries in Hilton Smith's fields. The going rate was a cent and a half per box, but I got one cent, since Hilton was feeding me and letting me stay at his home. In the better fields, we could pick 250 to 300 boxes a day. I was proud to be earning almost as much as the men working in the mines—for about two weeks, as long as the season lasted.

Next the blueberries ripened. I couldn't stay at Hilton's home because his wife was expecting a baby, so a couple of other boys and I stayed in a lean-to secured to a building on Everett Smith's property. We lived off the trout from a nearby stream, the generosity of a local poacher who shared his deer meat with us, and the farmers who gave us vegetables (to keep us from ransacking their gardens in the middle of the night). At the age of fifteen we were living completely on our own for the first time, and we cherished every minute of it.

A thirty-pound box of blueberries fetched fifty cents. The berries had to be clean, with no leaves or stems—clean enough to go directly into a pie shell. I was able to make a little more money than I had made picking strawberries, about three dollars a day, which was right on par with the miners. We used milk pails, filling one up from each kneeling-down position. We were not only bluenosers, we were blue-handed and blue-kneed too. With all of my savings from that summer, I was able to pay for my clothes and books for grade twelve in Amherst that fall.

At this age, you might be wondering about romance. Nowadays, kids are young when they begin to flirt. Back then, it was unheard of. We'd have lots of friends who were girls, but that was about it. I wasn't romantically interested in any of them. The most that ever happened was that we went skating together, and on occasion I'd walk a girl home. That was about the only time we'd ever hold hands.

But that didn't keep us from showing off. During blueberry time, we'd sit around in the evenings and crush fireflies so we could smear them on our shirts to make phosphorescent initials. Then we'd parade in front of the girls. How pleasant and simple life was in those days, and war was just around the corner.

I performed my first surgery during a hunting trip in Lynn Woods when I was fourteen. I was hunting for partridge, so I brought along the 20-gauge shotgun with some No. 6 shot. My good friend Gordie Bigelow had brought along his .22 rifle. He lagged behind me out of sight to go after a squirrel. I began to trail a rabbit; when I pulled the trigger, Gordie yelled. He had circled around me and had been hidden behind a thicket of bushes. I had shot the rabbit, but two pellets had ricocheted into Gordie's leg! One was close to the surface, so I went to work on it right away. I sterilized my hunting knife, extracted the pellet, and applied iodine from my first aid kit. The other was too deep, and it never did get removed. He carried it with him into the war and, much later, in 1988, into the grave.

I read whatever I could get my hands on, and especially enjoyed Horatio Alger books. I was inspired by the disadvantaged lad who, through hard work, succeeded and was able to motivate others. As for my own ambitions, they were simple. The mines didn't appeal to me—not because I was a snob, or because of the dangerous working conditions, or because the work was too hard. I just wanted to work full-time. That was my goal. I was raised to value work, and never considered welfare an option.

For grade twelve, I went off to Cumberland County Academy in Amherst. I lived and took my meals at Milton Flett's home, just across the road from the academy. Dad had been out of work due to sickness, so my grandmother paid the major expenses. Dad still managed to find seventy-five cents a week for me: twenty-five cents for the car ride to Amherst on Sunday nights, twenty-five cents for the ride to Springhill on Friday afternoons, and the balance was supposed to cover my school supplies, books, and countless incidentals. Luckily, I had my savings from the summer to supplement the remaining twenty-five cents.

Even though I had a full course load, including three different mathematics classes, chemistry, physics, science, English, French, and social studies, I went ahead and signed up for double-entry bookkeeping as well. This was offered after school hours at St. Charles Business College, so some days dragged on late. Even so, I was at the top of my class in bookkeeping, by no means an easy course. For the final exam, we had to set up a partnership business, write the cheques, find mistakes in a set of invoices, close the books after one month in business, do the trial balance, and divide the profits. All in one afternoon!

I made my first book in grade twelve, and it was homemade in every sense of the word. Our assignment was to compile an anthology of our favourite poems. Most of the class could afford to turn in lovely books with store-bought binders. I spent five cents on a writing pad, typed the poems with an old Oliver typewriter, and used India ink for the illustrations. Then I fashioned a cardboard cover and held it all together with black thread. The sixty-two-page booklet was certainly unique, and earned favourable remarks from the teacher.

During this time, the king and queen made their first visit to Canada. Springhill and Amherst area schoolchildren gathered to see the royal couple as they passed by on the train to Cape Tormentine on the way to Prince Edward Island. Les White and I were in charge of the grade one and two boys and were within a few feet of the king and queen on the observation platform at the back of the train. This was my first glimpse of royalty, and I received my first medallion on that occasion. After completing grade twelve, I decided to pursue accountancy back home, so I enrolled in a night school typing and shorthand class. I caught on to typing, but the shorthand eluded me. Writing it down was easy; reading it back was another matter! During the first test, most of the class quit writing in the middle, but I kept on faking it. I didn't notice I was the only one writing until the teacher's voice caught my attention. She was praising me! Then she asked me to read back what I had written. I turned beet red as I stared at the page of squiggly lines and mumbled, "Oh, are you supposed to read it back?"

After graduation I began to look for work. First I tried to get a job at a bank, but they turned me away on account of my height. At that time, tellers had to be tall enough to reach for a gun. I was five foot five and a half—one-half inch too short, so my career as a banker ended early.

Shortly afterwards, Lyman Austin, who ran a corner grocery near my home, made me an offer. He carried Rawleigh products—everything from medicines and salves to floor polish and vanilla extract—and wanted to set me loose selling door-to-door in the west end of town. I quickly established a schedule: show the merchandise and take orders during the week, and make deliveries and collect money on Saturdays, since Friday was pay-day at the mines. Lyman soon expanded my territory, so I came to know every family on that side of town, which amounted to about one-third of the population of Springhill.

I gave up Rawleigh products unexpectedly one day while shopping for my family at Leo Herrett's grocery store. Mr. Herrett offered me a full-time job, from eight o'clock in the morning until six o'clock at night, six days a week, for eight dollars a week. I began working at the grocery, and soon the bakers who supplied the store discovered that a pie or a cake for the clerks every now and again did wonders for sales.

A couple of months over sixteen, I was plenty old enough for a deer hunting licence, and so scraped up two dollars from my earnings. One October weekend, Pleaman and Steve Pyke and I went to Lynn Woods. Immediately, we saw the fresh deer tracks of a young buck pawing the ground. The Pykes walked on up ahead, and I stayed behind. I soon spotted a spike horn deer about fifty yards away, laying down in the bushes. As soon as he noticed me, he jumped up and I fired my single-shot 20-gauge shotgun, but he kept on going. By this time, my mouth was dry and my muscles tense. I had only fired at rabbits and partridge before. I said to myself, "My God, I hope I don't miss this. This is my first chance, I've got to get this." I was also thinking how nice it would be on the table. I was thinking all this at once as I loaded the second shell. I was leading the deer, and as I squeezed the trigger, I saw the big maple tree standing right smack in the way. Exasperated, I got another shell in, fired, and everything went quiet. I remember thinking, "How could I have missed that thing?" I scraped my foot on the ground to mark my spot, and walked over towards where I'd last seen the deer. There it was, lying on the ground. I was exhilarated.

I cut the deer's throat and dressed it. Thinking how difficult it had been for me to spend the two dollars on the licence, I laughed at myself. I wound up giving half of it to the Pykes, and then shared my half with my other friends. We were allowed two deer apiece that year, and I shot the second one later in the season in back of Thompson.

Art Booth's hunting camp was located halfway between Thompson and Atkinson, about eighteen miles from Springhill. Since I was the young fellow in the camp, everyone tried to con me into doing odd jobs by saying how handy I was. Peachie Wilson, who was always egging me on to cook, would compliment me on the tea. One morning, I got up and filled the teapot from the bog, an enlarged area in a nearby brook. After downing three cups, Peachie was singing the praises of the tea's flavour when something fell against his lip from the bottom of the cup. It was a tadpole that even had hind legs!

Every time I went out to the toilet at night, I carried my gun and a flashlight. Peachie would always kid me, saying, "Don't worry, the rabbits won't attack you!" One night it was Peachie's turn to go squat on the pole slung between the two trees and he went out with a flashlight, but no gun. He heard an animal coming towards him, which he assumed was a rabbit. When it reached his dangling feet, he turned the flashlight on. I heard two screams: first the wildcat, then Peachie. The next moment, Peachie came running in the tent with his pants halfway around his knees. After that, every time he went out to relieve himself at night, I would taunt him with, "Remember, Peachie, the rabbits won't attack you."

These hunting trips required backpacking, and in the days before sleeping bags, our packs were cumbersome. Sometimes they weighed upwards of one hundred pounds. I continued hunting right up until it was time to go overseas, and when I came back five years later, there were much fewer deer. I remember standing by the railway tracks and looking at the carcasses and bones left behind by illegal night hunters who had shot from the tracks and then couldn't locate the deer.

During my last year in school, I had joined but hadn't been able to take part in the Cadet Corps much, because of my studies. But I did make it to the inspection parade in the spring, and I took pride when I wore the kilt and regalia of the North Nova Scotia Highlanders.

The militia was active in Springhill at that time. On the weekends, we could see soldiers sending semaphore signals from the top of Victoria Street to the west side of town. In September, Neville Chamberlain, the prime minister of Great Britain, captured the headlines when he returned from Munich, Germany. As he faced the crowds in London, he waved the now-famous paper bearing Hitler's worthless signature, proclaiming, "Peace for our time." But Hitler's adventurism was about to discredit him. The Nazi troops marched into Poland, and World War Two began.

Some of the soldiers left Springhill right away, and the First Canadian Division soon went overseas. Our daily routine remained much as it had been—except for one thing: the mines began to work full-time. Coal was needed as fast as it could be produced, mostly to supply the trains and ships involved in the war effort. These were the days before diesel fuel, when coal was king. In fact, the Amherst recruiting office had a sign on the wall discouraging Springhill miners from enlisting. It said they could best serve the war effort by working in the mines.

Men were joining the army, navy, and air force, but I was still too young. Among the youngest in my graduating class, I was only two months over sixteen—a far cry from the minimum age of eighteen. Some of my schoolmates went overseas, and I can remember their letters describing German bombers and dogfights in the sky. We thrilled to read stories of the flotillas of tiny boats that braved the rough waters of the English Channel, the fury of the German air raids, and the bravery of both civilians and soldiers who sailed small watercraft to Dunkirk to rescue the stranded Allies. A Springhiller by the name of Tony Condy was the first Canadian to be decorated in World War Two, for getting his detachment of men out of France after the German invasion. Coincidentally, Harry Danson was the first Canadian serviceman to be decorated in World War One—also from Springhill.

My second lesson in surgery came at the grocery store as I watched the butchers cut up lamb and pig carcasses—first down the backbone, and then into the different cuts. Since there were no band saws in those days, they just had hand meat saws, cleavers, and butcher knives that we kept good and sharp. The meat cutters were expected to be able to cut a roast within an ounce of the customer's request, since money was scarce and there was no room for waste.

One day, I was in the shop while the meat cutters were on dinner break. A customer came in and asked for "undercut steak," which we now call filet mignon. None was already cut, but I knew the sides of beef were hanging in the freezer room. So I excused myself and went in to make the cut. I knew the undercut was next to the T-bone steaks, inside and near the top of the hind leg. And the meat cutter had explained to me exactly where to drive the knife through the hind quarter. As I was standing in the freezer room, slicing into a carcass for my first time, in walked my boss, Mr. Herrett.

"What the hell do you think you're doing?" he bellowed.

"Cutting some undercut," I muttered after a good hard swallow.

He stood there defiantly and said, "All right. Go ahead."

After watching me make the cut and then walk past him with a respectable-looking steak, he cleared his throat and went about his business.

A short time later, "Smokie" Martin (now Reverend Donald Martin) tried the same thing, but cut too far and ruined quite a few T-bone steaks. Mr. Herrett walked in on this fiasco, and the freezers had to work overtime to make up for the heat he gave Smokie. After that, Leo laid down the law. Absolutely no one was to cut into a side of beef except the meat cutters. And then he added, "...and Arnold, since he knows what he's doing." Shortly after this I put in for a raise, and wound up with an extra dollar a week.

As for surgery training, the meat cutting took me halfway there. Cutting things open is the first step; I learned how to put them back together much later in medical school.

The farm wagons and trucks were usually parked in back of the old post office. That meant we had to carry the groceries out of the store, across Main Street, and into the large parking lot where we'd search for the customer's vehicle. A ninety-eight-pound bag of flour on one shoulder and groceries in the other arm was standard. This was a bit of a strain, since I only weighed 110 pounds! And it got worse when the snow and ice were underfoot.

With the passing of New Year's Day, 1941, my life took a new tack, like a sailboat redirected by the wind. The next day I asked Leo for time off to join the army. He had no choice but to say yes. His parting words were, "Good luck, but you had better put some lead in your pockets." He knew I was underweight; to qualify, a recruit had to weigh 120 pounds. I was 10 pounds shy. My height problem at the bank was nothing compared to what lay ahead of me.

3. A Close Call at Sea

I HAD FIRST TRIED TO ENLIST WHEN THE NORTH NOVA SCOTIA HIGHLANDERS WERE RECRUITING IN THE SPRING OF 1940. I hitchhiked a ride on a motorcycle to Amherst and went through the medical exam all right—until I stepped onto the scale. I was ten pounds under, so I tried to convince the medical officer that I would soon put on weight.

Then he asked, "Are you sure you're nineteen?"

Someone laughed behind me when I answered, "Yes, sir." Sergeant Major Dennie Mackie had just been over to my home the night before, and he knew very well how old I was.

The medical officer spun right around and asked him my age. The Sergeant Major's "I don't rightly know, sir" put the skids to that enlistment.

The medical officer lit into me. "Get the hell out of here," he said, "and don't come back without a birth certificate." I was only seventeen at the time.

I figured my luck might change in another city, so a bunch of us drove to the air force recruiting centre in Moncton. A sign posted at the entrance read "DO NOT ENTER WITHOUT A BIRTH CERTIFICATE," so that was the end of round number two.

On January 2, 1941, I rode the evening train to Halifax for my third attempt. I had never been over fifty miles from home, and here I was going to a strange city with no idea where to put up for the night. I was anxious to join the army. Period. It was the thing to do in those days. We weren't interested in glory, or in becoming heroes, or anything like that. Our fathers had set the example in World War One, so we figured, it's here again and we've got to do our part. Plain and simple.

I was finally accepted in Halifax. Instead of reporting to the Cogswell Military Hospital as I was told to do, I said I would enlist at the Royal Canadian Army Medical Corps (RCAMC) in Aldershot. I got away with it since I hadn't signed any papers, and Aldershot happened to be recruiting at the time. I knew Aldershot would give me a much better shot at going overseas. When I signed my papers the next day, I became Private R. A. Burden, F84526, RCAMC, of the Aldershot Military Hospital. I'd be getting thirty cents a week less than I got at the grocery store, but I wouldn't have to look after my clothing, food, or housing. I was all set.

We never thought of the future—that we might get wounded or even killed. It was: "We're going through with this, and then we're coming back home." By the time the smoke lifted five years later, the truth had certainly drowned out our optimism. Thirty-three of the fifty-two Springhillers who had been my classmates in high school never returned.

I worked as a medical orderly in Aldershot for a few months. None of us knew much about hospital procedures so we groped through our jobs until they became familiar. Since there were no antibiotics at that time, a common procedure for an infected throat was to paint the inside tonsillar area and the back of the throat with argerol, a black liquid. One time I asked a fairly green orderly if he had done a throat-paint before.

He answered rather huffily, "I can certainly paint a throat."

So I turned him loose on a couple of patients. Hearing the laughter and commotion in the ward, I burst in. Two patients were sitting upright, their entire throats painted black on the outside. They had let him make a fool of himself, and the entire ward was benefitting.

Captain Bill Embree was a medical officer on one of the wards. He was posted to a draft that was proceeding overseas, so the other officers organized a party for him. He was very happy for the chance to join in the Allied war effort. His troop transport ship set sail for England, but he never arrived. A German submarine sank his ship in the Irish Sea. He and another officer made it to a lifeboat, but the submarine surfaced and sprayed it with machine-gun fire. We heard that Captain Embree was shot through the chest and went overboard. He was the first Canadian medical officer to be killed in the war.

Suddenly the tragedy of war struck me. It gave me pause, but my thinking about the future didn't change. Soldiers always tend to think, "There's only so many coming out—but I'm coming out."

Since I was in Aldershot from January to June, the extremes in temperature hammered me into condition. In the winter, the taxis from town only came as far as the main gate. We had to walk the rest of the way, so our ears and anything else that was exposed would freeze. Then, if the night-hut orderly had fallen asleep or gotten distracted from his responsibilities, the heat stove would be as cold as the doorknob. At minus-twenty-five Fahrenheit, a blanket did nothing for the chill. Then in the summertime, the combination of heat and dust turned the camp into a desert.

Just after my arrival at Aldershot I received my first—and last—handwritten letter from Dad. My stepmother always handled the correspondence. Even though he had a typewriter to transact business for the Legion, he wrote this one out longhand. He said he could have helped me out when I tried to enlist the first couple of times, but he preferred to let me make it on my own. He didn't want to interfere. He offered to back me up whenever I needed help, and gave the name of a close friend at Aldershot as someone I could count on if we went overseas. Then he gave me a word of advice from the first war: "On Parade—On Parade; Off Parade—Off Parade." I understood this to mean: Do what's ordered at the time, but don't try to pull rank. This was to come in handy in the years ahead. That letter made me feel ten feet tall—a rare and poignant expression from a man who often kept his feelings to himself.

After six weeks, I got forty-eight hours' leave. A buddy and I discovered the slowest train on earth—the one out of Kentville. First we had to wait until after midnight to catch the train to Windsor Junction. A milk run, it must have stopped to pick up cans at every farm along the way. Then we had to wait several hours in the station for the train to Truro. The cold stove in the station in the middle of February, with no wood or coal around, was not a welcome sight. After our threats to cut up the benches with the fire axe, the station master became more cooperative. At 7:00 AM we set off for Truro, waited some more, and then continued on to Springhill Junction, where we had to take a taxi home, arriving in mid-afternoon. It took fifteen hours to travel fifty miles, a hair over three miles an hour as the crow flies—and in this case, he was drunk.

I had the highest education in my unit at Aldershot, except for the officers. Thanks to my typing, shorthand, and bookkeeping I was soon transferred from ward orderly in the hospital to the administrative section of the orderly room of a military unit. I was delighted for the chance to develop my clerical and accountancy skills. I figured I'd never be able to go to college, so I looked to on-the-job training to prepare me for my future career.

After five months off requisite sundaes and banana splits at the canteen, I reached 120 pounds.

We had a short-tempered cook on the unit. One morning he slammed a pot on the stove and the alarm clock fell from its spot on the stove's warming closet into the soup pot. He was able to fish it out with a long fork, whereupon he doused it under the hot water tap and—miraculously—it survived. It was easy to start a riot in the kitchen after that. We'd just ask for some alarm-clock soup.

One day a letter came in from Debert requesting an orderly room clerk in the "A" category. By then I'd realized that Aldershot Military Hospital wouldn't be going overseas any time soon, so I decided to apply for this transfer. I was in "B" category, since I had been underweight when I enlisted. So I asked the commanding officer if I could have a medical exam to switch categories.

He snapped, "Get a medical officer to look after it and don't bother me."

I filled in the medical papers myself and "got a medical officer to sign them." Major Forbes's eyebrows raised up and he asked me how that medical officer could have signed while he was on leave.

I countered, "Well, he signed it in a hurry." He knew darn well I'd become proficient at signing the doctors' names on the charts. Even the doctors couldn't tell the difference between my forgeries and their own signatures.

He sucked in some air and said, "OK, I hope you're happy now."

"No, not exactly, sir. I've got another favour to ask," and I passed him a transfer to No. 7 Canadian General Hospital in Debert.

He looked it over and barked, "You tear this up and put up two stripes."

His offer to make me a corporal, lickety-split, made me think for a minute, but I answered, "No, I'm not interested in staying here. I enlisted to go overseas."

Then he coaxed me with Sergeant Nicholson's stripes, saying the sergeant was due for promotion in a month. When that didn't wash, he signed the papers. I passed up the chance to become sergeant after only a few months in the army because there was only one thing on my mind: going overseas.

Debert was a staging camp for transfers to Europe. I got to know the people I would be working with for the next four-and-a-half years. Major C. M. Bethune became the new registrar of the hospital shortly after my arrival, and remained in that position until just before the war's end. He received an Order of the British Empire (OBE) medal for his work as registrar for casualty handling in Europe, and after the war he went on to become chief administrator of the Victoria General Hospital in Halifax, where the nurses' residence was named after him.

Just before the North Nova Scotia Highlanders of the Third Canadian Division broke camp for overseas, their bagpipe band marched through the hospital for a final goodbye. The full bagpipe and drum band, with kettle, bass, and snare drums vibrated the corridor walls. It was a happy and sad occasion—happy because the pipe and drum music was so lively, and sad for those in hospital who had to stay behind. I found it extremely loud, with the walls ringing, but it was thrilling just the same.

I was both excited and relieved to board the *Andes*, a Caribbean cruise ship that had been stripped down to serve as a troop transport. Finally, the transatlantic crossing.

We were first instructed to find a hammock and hang it on a pair of hooks in the ceiling. Soon all the hooks were taken, and some of us had to improvise by hanging them above the toilets and over the tables. I wound up next to Glenn Palmer, who had worked with me in the orderly room, which was not the last time fate placed us together during the war.

It was November 11, 1941—hardly an ideal time to brave the North Atlantic. We sailed in a convoy of nine troop ships, which included the Fifth Canadian Armoured Division. After leaving the coast behind, we met up with our destroyer escorts. Imagine our surprise when we saw American flags flapping in the wind. This was before Pearl Harbour; the United States had not officially entered the war. But who were we to argue, as long as we had protection? Ours was the middle troop ship in three rows of three ships.

The snow and biting cold pummelled us on the open deck, and to make matters worse, we had to wear canvas shoes while on deck. After the first few minutes my feet were cold and wet, and they stayed that way for the entire voyage. We were dressed to kill in our greatcoats, mittens, scarves, Mae West life jackets, and in some cases, balaclavas and steel helmets. To warm up, we would stand toe to toe and pound each others' life jackets with our fists. This made us sweat, and then, of course, we'd cool off again. It's a wonder we didn't get pneumonia.

It was an ungodly trip. The food was horrible, fifty- to sixty-foot waves surrounded us a good part of the time, and we were dodging submarines all the way.

We nicknamed one of our sergeants "Sinbad the Sailor" because he had fancied himself a sailor before we left Halifax. He started getting seasick while we were still tied to the dock at Pier 21, and didn't improve much until we reached the other side.

During action stations, I was on duty at the ship's bow at a machine gun post. The rest of the time I worked in orderly room administration for our hospital, which handled the sick bay of the ship. Some men had broken bones from slipping on deck, but most were just plain seasick.

Ours was the biggest Canadian draft to go overseas at that time. It included the whole battalion of the Cape Breton Highlanders (one thousand men), the entire Fifth Canadian Division, and several other units the same size as ours.

Many of us who had Christmas parcels from home had to open them early...thanks to the unappetizing meals in the mess hall. On the way to our sleeping area we had to pass through the food galley, where the floor was always covered with sawdust and water. One day, a cook dressed in his dirty whites ambled through the doorway, struggling under the weight of a large metal tray of whole beef livers. One slipped off and fell on the floor just as I was passing him. He immediately picked it up, threw it on the table, sliced it, and tossed it into the cooking pan on the stove—dirt, sawdust, and all. I wondered who would be the lucky guy to get that one, and then hoped it would be an officer.

About a half hour later we were eating in the mess hall when another cook walked by, blowing his nose into the apron he was wearing. A few minutes later he came back carrying about a dozen loaves of oven-fresh bread out in front of him laying on the same apron. The fruit loaves and Christmas cookies our folks had given us for the holiday were gone before we reached shore.

Whenever there was the possibility of an attack by German forces, I was assigned as the first aid man for the crew on the machine gun post at the bow. One time I responded to the action station alert, which was in effect a loud siren. I was crossing the deck towards my post when I saw an American destroyer angling right in front of us so close I said to myself, "My God, we're going to cut that thing in two!" I reached out to brace myself and grabbed onto whatever was handy. I figured I was about to go for a very short swim in the ice-cold ocean.

And nothing happened! The destroyer went right by us. We were much higher up than the destroyer, which accounted for my misjudgment. Suddenly I heard and felt something I knew wasn't a deck gun. It felt like we'd run aground. I found out later that was when the destroyer dropped depth charges onto a German submarine, which had positioned itself between us and the next transport ship over.

The next day we were told that a German sub had been sunk. Action stations at the stern of the ship and the port side could see debris and oil that had blown up to the surface. The next day, Lord Haw-Haw, a German broadcaster, announced on international radio that the ship with No. 7 Canadian General Hospital aboard had been sunk. To this day, I don't know if my family ever heard that broadcast. That was my first close call.

After two long weeks we sighted Liverpool, England and everybody delighted at the prospect of quitting the ship. But then the *Andes* turned away and headed back into the Irish Sea. Our reaction is not printable, but the next morning when we sailed up to the docks at Liverpool, we saw animal carcasses and burnt timbers floating with the tide. We tied to the dock, which was still smoking from the previous night's bombing raid. I was beginning to understand the dangers of war.

We were billeted in the Canadian engineers' barracks in Cove, in the south of England. We didn't think much of the engineers, since the hot-water heating system wasn't working, and the toilets had backed up and wouldn't flush. We got in trouble for removing the blackout curtains from the doors and windows during the day and not getting them back up before nightfall. They were there to prevent the Germans from identifying targets in the dark.

After an uneventful stay there, we went to the village of Marston Green on the outskirts of Birmingham in the Midlands of England. We took over the military hospital there from No. 1 Canadian General Hospital. We were the only Canadian unit in the Midlands except for the air force, and they were scattered in small groups. After the hellish weather aboard ship we thrilled to see roses in bloom until Christmas, and our greatcoats remained on the rack for the rest of the winter.

The hospital compound was ringed by bomb craters of all sizes, but the Germans had not scored any direct hits on the camp itself. The hospital was surrounded by military installations and strategic targets, such as the BSA motorcycle factory ,which had been converted to manufacture machine guns, and an airplane factory that was turning out Sterling bombers.

When the air raids became our constant companions, we were busy looking after casualties. It still never occurred to me that I could become one of them.

On Christmas day, six of us went to the YMCA in Birmingham. We were told that British families would take us in for the holiday. When the other five had gone off with their hosts, I still sat there waiting. One of the organizers came out and told me my host had backed out, but suggested I wait a bit longer. Finally, Bea Brown showed up and took me on the train to her home in Solihull. I not only spent a heartwarming Christmas there, but many days afterwards. Bea and her relatives made me feel like one of the family. We got to reciprocate years later when the Commonwealth Air Training Plan sent British boys to Canada.

One of our strongest links with the villagers was our softball league. The orderly room staff, officers, nurses, orderlies, and service corps each had at least one team. Six or seven teams played every weekend. As we walked into Marston Green, the older women would poke their heads over their hedges to ask us which teams would be playing on Sunday afternoon, and who would be pitching. Most parts of England had not yet been introduced to baseball at that time. We came to feel almost like family members in the village, having stirred up interest in this foreign sport.

Baseball was in my blood. Dad had been a professional baseball player at one time, and was captain of the Springhill Fencebusters when they won the Nova Scotia and Maritime championships. His nickname was "Brownie."

As it turned out, Captain Ralph Fallow, a chaplain in my unit, had played ball with Brownie during World War One! One day the new recruits were playing the officers, and Captain Fallow was catching. It was my turn at bat. I connected with the ball and made it to first base, stole second, and then stole third due to an overthrow. The pitcher threw the ball to the captain at home plate, and he threw it back. I took off, and the captain stood in front of home plate to block me, but I didn't slide. I came in running, he went flying, and I was safe. I went up to him and said, "Are you hurt, sir?"

He shook his head and said, "I should have known better than to try that on Brownie Burden."

Two generations, two wars, and the same soldier. It made the world feel like a very small place.

After a few months in Marston Green, we were issued permanent passes as far away as Birmingham. As long as we didn't miss roll call or passive air defense (PAD) duty, we could come and go as we wished.

In March, mail caught up with us and I received a parcel and thirteen letters in the same day. We cherished anything from back home. The parcels contained things that were still plentiful in Canada but had already been rationed in England.

At that time, we were eating "bully beef"—canned beef from Argentina—practically three times a day. We would go into the mess hall and it would be sitting on our plates, still in the can. One day my buddy, Glenn Palmer, opened a letter from home and read that his folks had sent a parcel with something "he'd really enjoy." You should have seen Glenn's face when he pulled the wrapping off that parcel a few days later. It was a can of bully beef!

About this time, I began a correspondence course that was offered by the University of Toronto. I wanted to become an accountant after the war, so I took business English, arithmetic, and economics. Although I knew it could be several years, my future was in the back of my mind.

I rarely went to the dances at the village hall. Since I worked from 6:00 AM to 6:00 PM, I could have partied like a lot of the guys. One evening I was on my bicycle, and it was raining so hard I stopped off at the dance hall. Since I didn't know how to dance, everyone there decided it was time for me to learn. They didn't let me sit out a single dance that night. After 11:00 PM the rules limiting the size of the gathering went into effect. There could be no more than fifty assembled in one place, on account of the bombing. This was to limit the possible number of casualties per strike.

One day I took a bicycle ride to Coventry to the south. I wanted to visit the Anglican Church cathedral that had been bombed during the big raid on Coventry. Only the bell tower and the outside walls were left standing. With my five-dollar camera around my neck (which was just a hunk of plastic with a piece of glass in front), I climbed hundreds of circular steps up to the bell tower. I reached the top panting, and began to raise the camera to start shooting. At that moment, I was deafened by the huge bells. I got the hell out of there, with my head ringing as loud as the bells all the way down.

This was the first time church bells rang in England since the declaration of war. Early on, the decision was made to reserve the bells for announcing an invasion threat. But now that the threat was over, the church bells were ringing all over England—announcing the good news—at the same time they were assaulting my eardrums while I escaped the tower.

Two of the wards in our unit handled all of the chest and respiratory patients in the Canadian forces. Patients were shipped to us from Great Britain, Scotland, and northern Ireland before being sent back to Canada for discharge. Tuberculosis and pleurisy were the most common diseases. Once we became familiar with procedures, we were able to check 250 men through Admissions in less than three hours.

As orderly room clerks, we took advantage of the information at our fingertips. On night duty, when things were quiet, we'd telephone the girls in the Women's Auxiliary Air Force (WAAF) and make dates. That's how a lot of us got paired up, thanks to the telephone numbers we had of all the military installations in the area. Usually the girls would be on duty at barrage balloon sites. Cables were attached to big balloon that floated over the areas. These cables prevented the Germans from dive bombing or flying low. We'd arrange to meet the girls after their shifts.

April 7 was a beautiful, sunny day. I remember it because that was when the king's brother, the Duke of Kent, came to visit our hospital. I was picked as honour guard. After it was dismissed, I was off duty, and able to surprise him with my camera every time he stepped out of a ward into daylight. (Since I didn't have a flash, I had to wait outside to photograph him.) I was snapping photos left and right, and after several wards, he turned to the colonel and remarked in the most proper British accent, "Persistent chap, isn't he?" I wound up with about sixteen pictures. I felt honoured the duke would come to visit our unit. He was very down-to-earth as he walked along with the colonel and the matron of the unit. He visited all the patients, which numbered close to four hundred at that time.

We were all so sad to hear of his sudden death shortly afterwards when his plane crashed over Scotland.

In May of 1942 I got a pass to London and so took in the sights at Trafalgar Square, Hyde Park, the Tower of London, London Bridge, Westminster Abbey, and St. Paul's Cathedral. Within walking distance of Piccadilly Circus (which is not really a circus at all, but a circular road), I came upon the Windmill Theatre. The marquee bore the message: WE NEVER CLOSE. They remained open through all the bombing raids of the war. The Windmill's revue was a variety show, including comedy, music, singing, and chorus lines. As part of the show, there were live nude "statues" in alcoves along the walls. The women models remained absolutely motionless whenever the theatre was even slightly lit (which was most of the time), under penalty of law if they moved.

Madame Tussauds wax works museam was a must—I remembered Dad telling me about his frustrated conversation with a wax policeman during World War One. But since the Chamber of Horrors area had received a direct bomb strike, the wax works was not open to the public at that time.

Sometimes the differences between Canadian and British culture caught us off guard. A couple of privates were out walking two girls from Marston Green when they heard a door being pounded across the street. One of the girls remarked, "It's the Jones boys knocking up the Smith girls." They couldn't understand why our boys were doubled up with laughter. Both of the girls kept repeating the same thing, meaning that the boys were pounding on the girls' door to wake them up for work on the evening shift at the factory. They learned not to use that expression again around Canadian boys.

We used to spend a lot of time at a pub in the village. But one night it was invaded by a new lot of English lads from the Fleet Arm base a few miles away. It was crowded but friendly until one of them tripped one of us. Our fellow thought it was an accident, until the other one laughed. He then threw whatever ale hadn't spilled directly into the Englishman's face. Then two Fleet Arm lads grabbed our man while a third belted him. As you know, the Medical Corps is not usually a fighting unit. This was our first major engagement, and we rallied. We also won.

Luckily, the tavern keeper saw how it started, so he was on our side. The commanding officer of the Fleet Arm base told our colonel what injuries his boys had sustained, and how many had been admitted to sick bay. The colonel told him we were all on duty, so it couldn't have been his Medical Corps. The commanding officer left in disgust, and we got our pub back.

In early July we began to get regular air raids every night—sometimes three a night. On my next leave I went to Scotland and spent most of my time in Dunfermline, Andrew Carnegie's birthplace. After making his fortune in the United States, he didn't forget his homeland. He endowed the library and the museum in Pittencrieff Park. When I visited the museum, I saw a large tree trunk fossil by the main entrance. I was astonished to find out it had come from Joggins, Nova Scotia, about twenty-five miles from my hometown. It turns out that my uncle Bob used to work in the same office in Joggins as Mr. Bellmano, who sent the fossil to the Dumferline museum!

After the war, I found out that my uncle George, who had married Dad's sister, was born in Dunfermline. And little did I know that sixteen years later, I would receive the ribbon of the Carnegie Hero Award for my work during the Springhill Mine Disaster.

Tavelling through Scotland, the Scottish hospitality struck me as especially heartwarming. Jack Butler, a native of Dunfermline who had also lived in Toronto, greeted me on the street as soon as he spotted my uniform. "Hello, Canada!" he said, and then proceeded to drive me to the YMCA, where I enjoyed a hearty meal. Later he picked me up after work to take me to his home. He said, "If I tell my wife I've met a Canadian who I didn't bring home, she'd kick me!"

In Balloch, a French-Canadian sergeant and I stayed overnight in a hotel. Our plan was to catch the ferry up Loch Lomond at seven o'clock the next morning. In the lobby, we had noticed the sign "BREAKFAST AT 8:00," and so planned to go away hungry in the morning. At six o'clock the hotel staff roused us and told us to get dressed, that breakfast was almost ready. I didn't know it at the time, but I had discovered the land of my ancestors. The Lamonds (or Lamonts) hail from Dunfermline, and the Burdens are a sect of that clan.

4. Heavy Casualties

RETURNING FROM THAT LEAVE WAS LIKE WALKING FROM BROAD DAYLIGHT INTO THE PITCH-BLACK NIGHT. THE SECOND CANADIAN Division had landed in Dieppe, France, on August 19, 1942, and the casualties were extremely heavy. Making preparations to receive the wounded, the Canadian hospitals in the south of England had funnelled their patients to our unit. With all six hundred beds full, we learned that a trainload of battle casualties from Dieppe was heading our way.

We made room by moving one hundred patients to the recreation hall.

The men arrived with injuries from bomb blasts, machine guns, shrapnel, and mortar fire. Some were among the last soldiers evacuated off the beaches, and most required emergency surgery. Gas gangrene had set into many wounds, and without antibiotics, there was no choice but to amputate limbs. Six operating rooms worked all night, and by the next morning only one was permitted to remain open. The other five had become infected with germs from the gas gangrene.

That morning I was walking past the surgical operating room just as one of the garbage collectors fell over backwards in a faint. I rushed over to revive him and looking up from the ground, I saw the garbage can. Sticking straight up from a bed of bloody dressings was a blackened arm and hand. Perhaps the fellow saw the devil reaching up for him.

Despite the atrocious injuries from the Dieppe raid, I was proud that a Canadian division had been sent in on the first attempt to recapture France. Only about fifty Americans went in on that raid, most of whom never even saw the battlefield except from their posts aboard ship. Nevertheless, the Americans glorified themselves back home in the headlines: AMERICANS LAND IN FRANCE. I burned up when I heard this in light of the numbers of Canadian casualties being shipped in to our unit from Dieppe, and knowing that an entire Canadian division had spearheaded the attack.

On my way into London to deliver reports for the Canadian Military Headquarters, I ran into Chick Reedy on the Underground. I had known Chick since I was six years old. It was always a good feeling whenever I came across a Springhiller overseas.

Whether I was on leave or whether I was working at the hospital unit, I enjoyed myself. You might ask, "How could he enjoy working around casualties?" I was glad to be helping people. And besides, I was too busy to be depressed. The paperwork was important and I took pride in handling it accurately. After the war was over whoever survived battle wounds or illness would be qualified to receive military pensions, with the proper documentation. The admission slips we filled out ended up in Ottawa, and so the future of some of the patients depended on us.

After the Americans arrived in England, they challenged us to a baseball game, which the BBC dubbed "an international baseball game." They beat us five to four after fourteen innings.

We were in limbo as we turned the corner into 1943. The German invasion of England seemed unlikely, due to the build-up of Allied forces there, but the Allied invasion of Europe was still a distant plan. I received a letter from Gordie Bigelow informing me that he had come overseas with the air force and would be in London on landing leave. He had addressed it to the Canadian Army Overseas, since he didn't know where I was stationed in the British Isles. I asked the colonel for my leave and he said, "How do you expect to find him in London, one of the biggest cities in the world?" I explained how close Gordie and I had been, and he granted me nine days' leave.

I didn't doubt I could find him, but wasn't sure I could do it in the allotted time. Once in London, I made a beeline for the Beaver Club, a popular spot for Canadians in uniform. I wrote a notice for Gordie and left it pinned to the bulletin board. That evening I went to a dance and took in a show at the Whitehall Theatre, and the next morning, I'll be darned if I didn't walk right into Gordie at the club! He was with Frank Hunter and Eddie Weaver, also from Springhill. I had found him in less than a day and a half.

One evening Gordie and I planned to meet at the Windmill Theatre. As the hour approached, a heavy bombing raid was underway and the air raid sirens had begun to wail. The night was dark, the sky overcast with low, fast-moving clouds, as if even they were heading for a safe place. The narrow beams of the searchlights were splitting the sky wide open while the anti-aircraft shells blasted it with vivid yellow-orange explosions.

I crouched against the protecting wall of the theatre and listened to the whistle of bombs coming in above the crescendo of anti-aircraft fire. The high-explosive bombs fell some distance away, but incendiary bombs riddled the street right in front of me. Then a blazing incendiary dropped close to the wall. "Someone trying to keep the roof from catching fire," I figured. As I bent over to throw sandbags on the small bombs I had a tight feeling in my chest, and prayed that whoever was up there wouldn't throw one on my back. The sharp smell of smoke and burning asphalt lingered as the fires smouldered, the enemy engines faded away, and the all-clear sounded. Another raid was over. When Gordie showed up, I told him about the incendiaries, to which he replied, "Yes, that was me kicking them off the roof." As we headed into the variety show that never closed, I thought to myself, "That's what friends are for."

During another leave, I ran into Gordie again, this time with Ronnie Barrow and Reggie Calder. Another foursome from Springhill, and we had lots of news to exchange from back home. Each time we said goodbye to a fellow Springhiller, we knew it could be the last. In this case, Reg was killed two weeks later flying a Halifax bomber in a raid over Germany. Gordie was sent to the Mediterranean and only lived because of the favourable timing of his appendicitis. He was pulled off active duty and his replacement, along with his entire crew, was killed in a raid when their Lancaster bomber succumbed to enemy fire.

While he was still stationed at the Royal Canadian Air Force holding unit at Bournemouth, Gordie would come to visit me in Marston Green. We were each enjoying a glass of "haf and haf"[1] when the familiar cry of airraid sirens broke through the din around us—first from far away and then close by. Next came the stuttering clamour of engines overhead as enemy aircraft flew towards Birmingham, a few short miles away. I knew my hospital unit would be receiving casualties shortly, so we left the pub. As we headed into the darkness of the village, we could see the flickering red flashes of bombs falling on the city to the north, followed by the dancing flames of spreading fires. German planes that were caught by the cone of the searchlights exploded in the deadly delivery of anti-aircraft fire and spiralled to the ground.

We walked through a rain of shrapnel from anti-aircraft shells. A ten-foot-high fence butted up to the edge of the sidewalk before us. An electrical pole stood in our way and Gordie stepped ahead of me to get past it. The power pole had been covered by a white-painted tin band a few feet from the bottom, so it could be seen in the blackout. Suddenly, we heard a blast directly overhead, a piercing whistle, and a thud.

Gordie whipped around and said, "It's hit right behind us!"

I said, "Don't be so stupid. It's in front of us," and so we had something to argue about all the way back to the camp.

The next day on the way into Birmingham, we stopped cold at the power pole. A fist-sized piece of shrapnel was embedded in the metal band, chest high. It had whizzed right between us, and less than a foot from either of us. I guess the argument ended in a tie.

No. 5 Canadian General Hospital was moving on to Italy and so our unit broke camp and made our way through Bedding, Maidenhead, Kent, Taplow, and finally, to Cliveden. This was the site of a well-appointed hospital that had been built by the Canadian Red Cross on the estate, a quarter mile from the country mansion of the renowned Lord and Lady Astor. Swimming in the Thames River was a hop, skip, and a jump away—just a short walk through the woodlands.

Fleets of Canadian and British bombers roared overhead each night, and American Flying Forts[2] soared during the day. I was glad to see the Germans finally getting a dose of their own medicine. At night, I would look up into the sky and see squadrons of bombers forming up overhead. Since each bomber had four motors, there were four vapour trails per bomber. Hundreds of them produced a haze that blocked out the stars.

When we began preparations for our move into France, poison gas training was at the top of the list. One day, the training officers produced a dense concentration of tear gas mixed with smoke from smoke canisters. The wind changed abruptly and carried it towards the hospital, forcing some real life training among those who least needed it— a hundred lung cases in the chest wards! The patients, already short of breath, laboured with gas masks until exhaust fans dispersed the smoke.

On October 29, 1943, there was a party in honour of our commanding officer Colonel Halkett, who had just retired. The party was held at Cliveden House, Lord and Lady Astor's home. This had been the famous meeting place of literary and political leaders from all over the world. I marvelled over the guest book in the entry hall. It was a sizeable volume of hundreds of pages. Even though I knew Lady Astor had entertained nobility and heads of state, I was a bit shocked when I came across the signatures of Goering and Goebbels. Seeing their names scrawled in that distinguished album made me wonder about how fast things change.

The Cliveden estate was spectacular. Sunken gardens, finely manicured shrubberies, rhododendrons, rose bushes, and a rainbow of flowers adorned the grounds. Pheasants, rabbits, and partridge were everyday visitors.

A couple of the boys had had a few beers just before arriving at the party. Upon seeing a man in black tie and evening tails who they assumed was the butler, they asked for directions to the toilet. He said he was going there himself, so they followed. After some relief, they filtered into the main ballroom, and Lady Astor introduced her husband to the guests. The "butler" turned out to be Lord Astor.

In the interlude before the orchestra appeared, Major Tabbie Bethune played the piano, which was set off to one side of the dance floor. While turning the music pages for him, I noticed that everyone else was standing near the walls. When the orchestra set up and began to play, no one moved towards the dance floor. Suddenly I felt a hand tugging my arm. I looked up at Lady Astor. She commanded: "Let's get this shindig going!" We had the floor to ourselves that entire dance, and what a pair we made!...me in my clunky army boots and she in one of those floor-length dresses that looks as if a breath would blow it away. Either I somehow managed to keep off her feet or she adroitly steered clear of mine—probably both.

I had met her before at the hospital, during her visits to the patients. Whenever she came to the unit, one of us would have to carry the basket of freshly picked peaches from her garden, so that she could offer them to the bedridden. My most vivid memory of her was the time she visited a young Canadian soldier who was dying of tuberculosis. She said to him, "I hadn't expected to see you still alive." The patient gasped, and a funny look came over his face. A hush fell over the ward, and she damn near would have gotten the rest of the peaches on her head if I had been holding the basket. The patient only lived a week or so afterwards.

We soon found out that the Third Canadian Division and the Fifty-first Highland Division would be among the first troops to land on D-Day, and that our unit would be the first Canadian hospital to land in France after D-Day.

At this time I was paraded before the colonel, who asked if I would go back to Canada for officer training. I refused promotion once again, this time so that I could continue with my unit and go into France on the invasion.

George Morris from Springhill had been in our hospital for over a month. One evening, Major Charlie Jones came into Admitting and Discharge waving an X-ray film, yelling, "Where the hell is that goddamned Springhiller?"

I said, "There are four or five of us, Major, which did you want to see?"

He shot back, "George Morris. I threw him out of the army in Canada with silicosis and I'm going to throw him out again." George was on the next convoy back to Canada.

He and another miner by the name of John Sheepwash had contracted silicosis drilling stone tunnels in the soft coal mines in Springhill, but the Nova Scotia Workmen's Compensation Board did not recognize it as a compensable injury. Stone carvers and other tradesmen received compensation for silicosis, but at that time miners did not. Through the efforts of these two men, in concert with the Springhill branch of the Royal Canadian Legion, silicosis from working in soft coal mines was finally recognized as compensable. Dad was secretary of the Legion at that time and was one of many who pushed for this legislation.

On January 16, 1944, I was paraded before Colonel Victor Mader, who asked if I had a bicycle. Of course he knew I did, and I was puzzled by his question, but I promptly answered in the affirmative. Then I noticed the sidearms on Major Jones, who was standing beside me in the colonel's office. I knew something unusual was taking place, because medical officers only wear sidearms when they're in action in order to protect patients. So my curiosity was piqued.

The colonel said, "Drive your bicycle along with Major Jones to the [train] station. If you can get a train to London, that's fine. If not, you'll have to ride the bicycles all the way into London." The fog that day was so dense that motorcycles, dispatch riders, and cars were immobilized. Trains were questionable. I did not relish the fifty-mile ride to London, but made ready for the journey.

"Stay with Major Jones at all times," the colonel instructed me. "If he has to go to the toilet, stand outside the door so you can see his feet. You must not let him out of your sight until you reach CMHQ (Canadian Military Headquarters) in London."

This was the first time I had received that type of order, and I became even more curious about our mission. The two of us set out for the station, and sure enough, a train had just arrived. Due to the fog, it was twenty-four hours late! So instead of fifty miles of pedalling, it was only one and a half. Major Jones had an envoy case strapped to his arm, secured by a locked chain. Even he didn't have the key—that was with one of the senior officers of our unit. He delivered the documents without incident, and it was only later that I realized what they were—our unit's invasion plans after D-Day.

Not long afterwards, on March 7, each of us in the unit was awarded our first medal—the Canadian Voluntary Service Medal and Clasp. The first time I wore my medal ribbon I went into London on leave. That night there was a heavy firebombing raid in the city, and when I went to inspect the damage the next morning, the street itself was on fire. Instead of cobblestones, there were tar-soaked blocks of wood the size of bricks that had been set in the road end to end, and they were still smouldering.

At Helmsley, a small town in Yorkshire, we began intensive training for our entry into France after D-Day. We simulated field conditions on the continent by practicing field cooking, setting up tents, sleeping on the ground, learning how to keep our kits dry, and digging makeshift latrines. We sterilized water in tanker trucks as well as in our own water bottles, went on route marches, and lived in our small tent city for about a month.

We discovered the North Nova Scotia Highlanders were less than two miles away, and so we met with friends and relations whom we hadn't seen since Camberley in the south of England in 1941. That was the last time we saw many of them, since hundreds were killed on D-Day, plus two at Authie and Buron, and more in later battles in France.

There were a few replacement men in our unit, who were on hand to take the place of the men who weren't medically fit. One of these was a heavy-set chap from Ontario. He was checked into the tent next to mine, along with some of the orderly room staff. I never got to know him. He had only been there one day when the rest of us were going off to see the movie *Commandos Strike At Dawn*. We went in to his tent to invite him along. He was busily sharpening his five-inch utility knife and didn't even look up. Our bantering back and forth didn't spark his attention; he was reticent as he declined our offer, pulling his blade across the stone all the while.

When we got back later that night, we were standing outside his tent, making small talk. One of the guys heard a gurgling sound, and we rushed in. The service knife was on the floor beside his hand, with the sharp edge facing us. He was gasping in a pool of blood. His throat was slit. Blood clung to the tent walls. We were too late; in a few moments, he died. I remember standing there motionless while one thought stabbed my brain: "Why would somebody do this?" Later I wondered, "If he's afraid of getting shot in France, why kill himself in England to prevent it?" No one had any answers—he was another war casualty.

All of our packs were the same size, and the bigger fellows had a terrible time cramming everything into theirs, especially their oversized shoes. Someone with a black sense of humour remarked that this fellow's shoes must have been too big to go into his packs.

Our unit moved to Eastbourne, on the south coast of England. A raging storm over the channel kept us from sailing immediately to France. It was a heavy summer storm—almost a hurricane. From the windows of the South Cliffe Hotel, we had a great view of the v-1 rockets exploding into the sea. Every time a bomb dropped, a shock wave would come towards the hotel. Above the wave appeared a thicker column of air, which was in fact compressed air from the bomb blast. Some of the v-1 rockets, which were nicknamed "doodlebugs," were so low that the boys said they could hit them with a broom from the rooftop—but no one tried.

The Tempest fighter planes would dive down and insert the tips of their wings under the wings of the v-1 rockets. This would upset the gyrocompass, causing the v-1s to crash. One Tempest malfunctioned and landed in the sea in front of us. We watched an air/sea rescue boat make it to the plane within minutes. The pilot crossed the wing of his sinking plane and jumped into the boat without even getting his feet wet. The next day, the newspapers trumpeted this as the fastest air/sea rescue ever made.

Since D-Day had already begun on June 6, the action was intense on land, sea, and air. Sixteen days after D-Day we had our last decent meal and boarded the *Liberty* ship, which sailed eastward for the coast of France. Early the next morning, still a long ways from France, we were told to disembark onto an assault landing craft (ALC). I was in full battledress, carrying all my equipment: gas mask, ground sheet, gas cape, and rolled-up blanket were all piled on top of a forty-pound pack. A quart water bottle hung from my webbing, and a small pack strapped to my side held forty-eight hours' worth of rations, shaving gear, socks, and other incidentals. Each of us laboured under the weight, climbing down the cargo nets in full marching order. But when I stuck out my foot, the landing craft wasn't there—it was twenty feet below. Another close call. Both vessels were alternately moving forward and sideways, and had we let go too soon or too late, we would have missed the landing craft as it bobbed up and down in the twenty-foot seas.

When we landed at Arromanches we were told to get off the beach on the double, and to stay between the tapes since the mines hadn't yet been cleared. We marched inland. A German plane, an ME 109, machine-gunned us in an open field before getting shot down and exploding in the next field over. The pilot floated over our heads in a parachute.

A truck convoy took us seven miles inland and dumped us off in a field. There were ready-made slit trenches, but we had to kick the you-know-what out of them before bedding down for the night, since the previous occupants had relieved themselves before moving on. It was a noisy night, with naval ships firing broadsides overhead.

About ten miles from where we landed, we set up our hospital on the outskirts of Bayeaux. The rations we were issued in England kept us going the first couple of days, but they were far from appetizing: dried oatmeal, hardtack, and compressed "food" that nobody could identify. We found some potatoes the size of marbles in an open field, which we rubbed clean and ate raw.

The officers searched along the fifteen-mile Canadian beachhead for all the hospital equipment—100 ten ton trucks' worth. Shortly afterwards, once we had set up the tent hospital, the incoming convoys of casualties were especially heavy. We worked non-stop. At one point Major Bethune came in and asked for my cup and mess tins. This seemed like a strange request, but I quickly obliged. He took them over to his tent, filled them with food, and invited me to eat at his place. Again, this was compo rations—compressed "food"—and although I had no idea what I was eating, it was nutritious and left me with a full stomach. He then proceeded to feed the rest of the admitting staff.

Ten to fifteen miles away, the fighting at the Carpriquet Airport, Falaise Gap, and Caen was intense. The Falaise Gap was the spot where a German army was trapped after the Canadian and British forces attacked the Germans at Caen and Falaise and demolished the bridges over the nearby rivers. The First Polish Armoured Division had joined the Canadian and British troops there, and we were admitting up to four hundred casualties a day. The First Polish Armour attacked the well dug-in Germans in their hull-down position, with only their gun turrets above ground. This may have been in retaliation for Warsaw, but they were no match for the fortified German tanks. The Poles suffered very severe burns when they bailed out of their flaming tanks, and then caught the brunt of German aggression: rifle and machine-gun fire.

For a few days we saw nothing but severe burn cases complicated by bullet wounds. The admitting tent stank of burnt flesh and scorched uniforms. Some of the casualties lay on stretchers with intravenous plasma running into one arm and a penicillin drip into a vein in the other. When the stretchers were moved, the injured moaned and stared at us with frightened eyes and ghost-like faces, still in shock. These were some of the heaviest casualties I saw overseas. We sealifted up to four hundred a day back to England, for a daily turnover of eight hundred soldiers. Later, when the Allies gained more territory, metal mesh was laid down in a field to improvise a landing strip. Then we were able to move casualties out by both sea and air. On one occasion I didn't make it back to my tent for five days to clean up, shave, or change clothes. We just dropped down onto stretchers until the next convoy arrived. At midnight each night I typed six copies of all admissions, discharges, the seriously ill, dangerously ill, and deaths over the preceding twenty-four-hour period.

After the heavy Polish casualties the shoe was soon on the other foot. Our twenty-five-pounder guns and howitzers on the ground, in combination with the Tempests, Spitfires, and other planes bombing and machine-gunning from the air, inflicted a severe punishment on the Germans. Then we began to see Germans who had such extensive battle shock and concussions from bomb blasts that they would crawl under stretchers at the slightest unexpected sound in the admitting tent, such as a metal cup falling off a table onto the canvas floor. Battle shock took different forms. Some of the soldiers went blind after seeing their friends getting their heads blown off. The Allied forces had finally broken out from their beachhead positions, and were now on their way to liberate Europe.

One night Glenn Palmer and I were on duty in the admission tent. Suddenly anti-aircraft gun blasts sounded, followed by the screeching sound of a German Stuka dive-bomber and the unmistakable whistle of an incoming bomb. I dove under the table and Glenn took off up the road just before the thud. "Oh no, not a delayed action bomb," I thought as I huddled in fright. There was nothing to do but wait for it to explode, and it was too close for comfort.

Glenn came back in with blood running from his chin and elbows, and down his legs. "It's not from the bomb," he said, shaken. "You know where they're fixing the road? I ran into the piled debris."

There wasn't much I could do to help; I just laughed at him. The next morning we searched for the bomb that never went off. The joke was on us when we found a shell cap from an anti-aircraft shell that had been fired at the plane.

There was a new military cemetery nearby with just a few white wooden crosses. A couple of months after the breakout of the bridgehead, it had become thick with crosses and populated with the war dead.

On D-Day plus two, the North Nova Scotia Highlanders' battalion had spread out between Authie and Buron. The Germans attacked with tanks and infantry, and the North Novas put up such a good fight that they stopped a German corps[4] under General Kurt Meyer. Finally some of the North Novas had to surrender when they ran out of ammunition. With very little back up support, and no heavy gun support, they succeeded in stopping the Germans from advancing to the beachhead. Had the Germans made it to the beachhead, they could have divided the remaining Canadian and British forces to subvert the Allied advance.

The Hitler Youth Regiment had murdered twenty-seven North Nova Scotia Highlanders—mostly Cape Bretoners— whom they had captured at Authie and Buron on D-Day plus two. Hitler's boys tied their hands behind their backs, machine-gunned them, and then proceeded to drive over them with tanks. I heard this report from an eyewitness. Another group from C Company of the North Novas barely escaped the same fate. The Youth Regiment had mounted the machine guns and were ready to fire when a German sergeant ran out of a tent screaming, "Schiess nicht! Schiess nicht!"[5] The murder of these twenty-seven men constituted at least part of the reason the German general Kurt Meyer was tried for war crimes and spent time in the Canadian prison in Dorchester, New Brunswick, after the war.

One day, several of us were walking along the main highway away from Bayeux and came upon a French woman milking a cow. With the best grammar I could muster, I asked: "Avez-vous vendre du lait?" to which she replied, "Bientot." None of us remembered what this meant, not even a Frenchman from Cape Breton! We finally realized that she was asking if we could wait until she was through milking. It tasted divine after our steady diet of dried food, compo rations, and water.

Occasionally we got a break. One time we took a truck to the section of the beachhead that had been cleared of mines. We went swimming out among the obstacles that had been placed to sink the landing craft. We gallivanted in the water as the sun baked down on us. When we came ashore, our legs were shiny black up to our knees. A thick layer of bunker fuel oil lay under-water. We had to douse ourselves with gasoline to clean up. I lay down in the sand to catch some sun. As I ran my fingers through the sand, I found some fingers that weren't mine—a graphic reminder that not long ago this beach had been a battleground.

The army newspaper, the *Mapleleaf*, was published for the first time in France. About this time a fellow on a motorcycle drove up and handed me a bundle of Vol. I, No. 1 to distribute to our unit. I still have my copy.

After the breakout of the beachhead, the armies moved north, so we broke camp and relocated just inland from Dieppe. As we moved through Caen, all I could do was stare at the wreckage that had been left by the thousand-bomber raid that had been conducted while we were in Bayeux. Houses were smashed, streets were devastated, and even the course of the river had been changed. The bombing had plugged the Orne River, forcing the water to reverse its flow. The downtown core was in shambles. Caen, which had been the focal point of the German command, had been decimated by over ten thousand tons of explosives.

As the bombers flew over our camp their multiple heavy motors would shake the ground. Some of the planes flew so low that we could actually see the bombs in the open bomb-bay doors. We hoped the bomb aimers didn't have hay fever. We didn't want them to sneeze while passing overhead.

NOTES

1. Haf and haf: Half light ale and half dark ale.

2. Flying Forts: B52 bombers.

3. Breakout of a bridgehead: Funneling out of troops after a major attack.

4. German corps: Approximately 27,000 men.

5. "Schiess nicht! Schiess nicht!": "Don't shoot! Don't shoot!"

5. Sandbostel Concentration Camp

AFTER CAEN, WE MOVED INTO THE VILLAGE OF ARQUES-LA-BATAILLE, JUST INLAND FROM DIEPPE. AS SOON AS WE COULD get passes, we went into the city to see the beaches. The gun emplacements covered the entire beach area, and I wondered how anyone could have escaped alive in 1942. I shot my last roll of film and headed straight for a photo shop in town. I was able to buy some outdated film and a few filters that had been hidden from the Germans. But the grand prize was a series of eight photos that had been taken just after the Dieppe raid. A German officer had brought them in for processing, and the enterprising shopkeeper had made copies of the negatives for his own purposes. He gave me a set for my collection.

One photo shows a dead American soldier lying on the beach with the Churchill tanks of the Calgary Highlanders still burning. A landing craft is on fire in the foreground, as are a tobacco factory and industrial buildings in the distance. Another photo shows Canadian prisoners being marched through the streets of Dieppe with their hands on their heads.

Even though the battlefront had moved forward, it left behind delayed reactions. At Arques-la-Bataille, a manhole cover lay at the juncture of a Y in the road. This was a busy thoroughfare: ambulance convoys, tanks, leave trucks, and general traffic passed over it daily. Weeks later, a Jeep running over the manhole detonated a pressure mine that had been placed just underneath the cover, and the truck blew up.

One beautiful sunny day when I was off duty, I was wandering around with my camera and had cut across the fields to take some pictures of the ruins of the old Arques castle. Birds were singing and chasing insects in the grass, and wildflowers were on the way; it was a fabulous day to be alive. As I neared the ruins, I saw a Frenchman down on the road waving his arms over his head and yelling, but I couldn't make out what he was saying. Since I wasn't causing any trouble, I kept going on my merry way. There was an archway in the stone ruins, and a galloping horse had been fashioned in the stone above the arch. It made an excellent photograph. Once I was satisfied with my pictures, I ambled nonchalantly to where the farmer was standing. He didn't say a word, just shook his head and pointed to a sign by the roadside: "Minen." I had been walking in a German minefield.

After we were in France a short time, our unit got parts from two trucks that had been damaged, and from them we made one. We painted it with our insignia and used it for unofficial business.

One evening Glenn and I took the truck into Dieppe to see a movie. At that time, all vehicles had to be immobilized, so Glenn removed the gas pedal linkage, since he couldn't get to the rotor button. While we were in the movie, the Provost Corps confiscated the truck, using the hand throttle. They drove it into their compound, which was surrounded by barbed wire and protected by an armed guard at the gate.

Glenn and I figured we'd take our chances, so I went up to the compound as a decoy. I acted drunk and the guard got such a kick out of the dumb guy who couldn't find his way back to his unit that Glenn walked right in behind him, put the linkage back in the truck, and drove out. I jumped onto the running board and away we went.

The next day the provost marshall came to see our registrar, Major Tabbie Bethune. Tabbie was in on our escapade. The provost marshall addressed him stiffly: "I want to arrest the men that stole the truck."

"What truck, and what marking did it have?"

The provost marshall replied, "It had the markings of No. 7 Canadian General Hospital."

"Oh," Tabbie said slowly. "You want us to arrest the provost men that stole our truck?"

Their conversation tapered off quickly at that point. The provost marshall was almost in tears when he left. Our truck was safe after that episode, and Glenn and I congratulated each other on our daredevil mission.

It's amazing that our outfit landed back home intact. We suffered injuries, but no deaths. We were bombed in England and strafed on the shore; we had rockets land in our camp and mines blow up around us. And when it was time to resume our lives in Canada, every last one of us returned.

In late October and November, the river started to freeze over. We were still in tents; the wind grew fierce, especially when it rained. The nurses were staying at Chateau St. Clair, and the admitting department was finally moved to Chateau Martigny. Glenn and I were on duty the first night and had to find wood for the fireplace. There were no forests in sight, just logs stuck into the ground in the adjacent field to ward off glider landings. Since it was dark, we worried that the logs could be mined. Two dozen German prisoners of war were being housed on the second floor, but there was nowhere to send them foraging.

Glenn walked out with a fire axe and came back in with a bundle of lovely dry wood. Nobody asked questions, and we stayed warm all night. The next morning, a Frenchwoman came to the door flailing her arms and talking so fast we couldn't make out a word. Finally we got her to slow down. It turned out that something was missing—the hitching rack in front of the chateau. It was a historic monument because Napoleon had tied his horse there! Instead, there were wood chips scattered on the ground. After taking in a few sheepish grins and one or two scratched heads, she threw up her hands and set off in search of the colonel.

Glenn and I were still sleeping on the ground, and so had to fend for ourselves. We pounded stakes into the ground and stretched burlap bags across the stakes to elevate us about two feet from the cold earth. Before going to bed, we'd close the tent flaps and crank up the kerosene heater we had "borrowed" from the hospital. First we'd work up a sweat before getting undressed, and then we'd take off our pants and put them on the burlap under us to press them while we slept. We used our tunics for pillows. But the sweat would freeze our hair to the tunics by morning. After thawing it from our faces, we would get dressed, go down to the river, and break ice to wash before going to breakfast. The last thing we would do before leaving the breakfast tent was get a hot cup of tea or coffee, and rush to our tent to shave while it was still warm.

Finally, it got too cold to maintain battle casualties in tents. Even attempts to heat them with kerosene failed. We had between two and three hundred sick and injured personnel at that time. The war was advancing from France to Belgium, and so we broke camp and headed for Turnhout, Belgium.

We were billeted in St. Joseph's College, a Jesuit college that the Germans had confiscated just after Dunkirk to house the Luftwaffe[1]. The ceiling in the recreation room was twenty-five feet high and on one of the walls was a huge mural of a dog-fight—with the German planes winning, of course. It was a four-storey building with plenty of room for the patients as well as our whole unit.

Before the British took Turnhout, the White Brigade had been quite active in the town. When we arrived, they came to offer help and wound up carrying stretchers for us. They were not run-of-the-mill townspeople. One of them was studying six languages, another owned a playing card factory, a third was a diamond merchant. One day he came in carefully holding a handkerchief folded over. It contained a dozen or so large diamonds he wanted to show us.

And then there was Jos Vogels. Jos was about forty-five years old, and he only spoke Flemish. Our conversations were patch-works of sign language, French, English, and German, but we were able to understand one another. He belonged to the White Brigade. He worked for the telephone company as an engineer, and managed to subvert the German communications network almost single-handedly. He would dig a lot of holes over the buried telephone cables between the cities so that, at a given time, all the cables could be cut in one synchronized operation and then immediately filled with dirt. It would take the Germans a long time to make repairs, during which time Jos and the White Brigade would be cutting more cables or digging further holes. Finally the Gestapo figured it had to be a telephone engineer, and they appeared at his front door. Jos slipped out the back, and over the ensuing months his family worried that he had been captured or killed.

Five and a half months later, Jos turned up sitting on the front of a British tank as he guided the British into Turnhout and towards the German targets. Among the war mementos I treasure the most are the arm band and badge he gave me.

Jos invited me to his home one afternoon. This promised to be challenging since we would have to rely on our bastardization of German, French, Dutch, and Flemish to understand one another, because his true and only language was Flemish.

His married daughter, her husband, their two children, and another daughter were there to greet us. When it came time to eat, only Jos and I sat down to the dining table covered in the finest linen and set with fancy china—and of course Belgian crystal. I grew more and more uncomfortable as the others sat back and watched. Jos's daughters took turns serving. A plate of vegetables—mostly potatoes—was set down between us, and there was not really enough there for two. After spooning potatoes onto my plate, I caught on from Jos: we were both to eat out of that plate directly, a forkful at a time.

Next, the young daughter served a piece of steak onto my plate, about one-half inch thick and two and a half inches around. The children, aged ten and three, were eyeing every mouthful, which made me realize that this was probably a lot of their ration. I could almost hear them thinking: "Is he going to eat it all, or is he going to leave us some?" To be a good guest, I had to eat it all. Later I found out that this meal amounted to one week's ration for the entire family.

At the same time, they all appreciated having a liberator—a Canadian soldier—in their home. Even the three-year-old knew what it had been like under the tyranny of the Germans, since grandfather had suddenly vanished while the Gestapo were banging on the front door. So it was mixed: while appreciating me, they also wished I wouldn't eat all of their food!

The following day, I took some cigarettes to the cook in our unit.

"I'd like some meat," I said.

"I can't give it to you," he replied curtly.

"I've got some cigarettes here," I countered, and then explained what I wanted it for.

"You keep the cigarettes. I'll get you some meat," he said and went back to the freezer. A few minutes later he came out with a twenty-pound roast. I wrapped it up in brown paper and kept it handy until Jos was ready to go home that day. As I handed it to him, I warned, "Don't open this until you get home."

Afterwards he kept telling me how much that meant to his family—of course, not when the other stretcher-bearers were within earshot.

Just before Christmas, our Belgian friends became exceptionally tidy. They picked up every gum wrapper, cigarette package, and piece of cardboard. The grounds and admitting room were immaculate, and only on Christmas morning did we find out why. Jos and company came into our unit carrying a spruce Christmas tree about three and a half feet tall. If was fully decorated with ornaments made from tinsel, cotton, gum wrappers, and whatever else they found on the ground. A star crowned the top and ball ornaments hung from the limbs. To make the star, they had covered a cardboard cut-out with gum wrapper foil.

They came in carrying a box of apples and pears, singing "Silent Night" in French, English, Flemish, and German. That was a very poignant moment for me. I felt lonely and homesick, on my fourth year away. At the same time, I was touched by this group of men doing something for us, a bunch of foreigners. And knowing how little food they had for rationing, this was an expression of great generosity.

One evening I was in the yard of the hospital when I saw a v-1 rocket pass directly over my head, right on course for the hospital. As I dove into the mud, I thought, "There goes about three hundred patients along with the entire unit." v-1s carried a ton of high explosives. But there was no explosion. "Thank God" was my first impression until I looked around. The rocket had gone over the building but was now on an elliptical course, and getting lower. I ran in the opposite direction of the probable blast and dove into the mud again. Again it was high, so I didn't waste any time running further from the building. I hit the mud a third time as the rocket exploded overhead. It could have been disastrous for No. 7 Canadian General Hospital. Instead, one admitting clerk was covered with mud.

Later on, a v-2 rocket landed in the middle of the camp. Luckily, it hit soft ground as it came down from its sixty-mile altitude, and the explosion mushroomed over the camp, causing only minimal damage. It tore out windows and door frames a bit further away. Guess we were meant to come back from the war.

On September 17, 1944, the operation of "Market Garden" took place at Arnhem with thousands of planes and gliders.

We handled casualties from the operation, which was immortalized in the book, and later the movie, *A Bridge Too Far*.

After some weeks of quiet, the Germans broke through the American lines in the Ardennes between Belgium and France. This was a heavily wooded area south of our position. We were awakened at about 6:00 AM with orders to evacuate our patients to the hospitals in Brussels, and to pack up in order to move out by noon. A Canadian division and a Scottish division were to attack the German spearhead from the side, and we were to move along with them to handle the casualties. When that didn't happen, we were told to reopen and receive the patients from the 1,200-bed No. 10 Canadian Hospital that had also been located in Turnhout. The generals decided to pull No. 10 out and leave us there. The boys who had difficulty adapting to changing conditions had trouble that day, especially since we had been told to get rid of all the German souvenirs we had collected in anticipation of a German incursion. At this time, we saw our first-ever German jet fighter plane.

When things died down, I was out taking pictures on the outskirts of the city. I came upon a windmill and saw a Canadian soldier there, admiring it. It was Irwin MacEachern who I've known since I was five! He grew up seven houses down from me in the next block back home. The miller obligingly took my camera and snapped a few souvenir pictures of us.

Travelling by truck convoy some months later, we crossed a long Bailey bridge that spanned the Rhine River. It was time to follow our forces into Germany. The Canadian army swung to the left for the liberation of Holland, but we went with the 51st Highland Division and the 1st British Armoured Division, which were intent on capturing the German naval ports on the North Sea. The first thing we saw was a large sign posted to one side of the road:

ENTERING GERMANY
BE ON YOUR GUARD
DON'T FRATERNIZE WITH GERMANS.

As we moved into the area, a tank battle was in progress. The tanks were on opposite sides of the river in Bremen. Years later, Steve Pyke, who had been a navigator in the Royal Canadian Air Force during the war, showed me a map of his last bombing mission: the war over Bremen in 1944. He flew a Halifax bomber in that raid. He said they were told not to drop the bombs if they couldn't identify the river. Since there was a thick cloud cover, they later discharged the bombs into the sea. I said, "Thanks," since we were the troops on the other side of the river who would have been blown up had the bombers misjudged their targets.

Imagine being killed in Germany during the war by your own next door neighbour from Springhill!

We came to one bombed German town after another. We were relieved to see such massive damage in enemy territory. Buildings were in ruins, towns had been smashed down flat. We had seen villages, schools, and non-military areas in England and France badly hit, and now it was nice to see that Germany had suffered some of the same. Nevertheless, it was always sad to see civilian casualties, whether they were friend or enemy.

In Bassum, we settled in a German hospital that had been used by the Germans as a maternity hospital for the unwed mothers who were charged with the responsibility to carry on the Aryan race. Soon casualties coming into our unit fell off— from one hundred a day to fifty a day, and then less. The troops couldn't tell where the Germans had retreated. We wondered why our troops weren't moving into Berlin, and later found that the politicians let the Russians take it instead.

Sandbostel concentration camp—not a well-known name, except for those who managed to escape its horrors alive—was liberated, and we saw our first German death camp. We had not heard of Bergen-Belsen, Buchenwald, and the others at that time. The inmates of this camp were mainly political prisoners, but there were also Canadians who had been in there a short time, captured in the Dieppe raid. Railcars sat in the yard with full loads of corpses stacked like cordwood. When the camp was liberated by our conquering armies, we began to admit those who were still alive by the hundreds. Our hatred of the Germans reached new heights. The inmates were emaciated. Six-foot men weighed sixty or seventy pounds. Their eyes were wide open windows of misery, staring almost as if not seeing. Their skin was sallow and broken into sores, and those who could stand upright walked with a shuffling gait. Many were afflicted with nervous disorders. Their skin was so tightly stretched, bones seemed on the verge of poking through. You just saw the eyes and the heads.

These scrawny bodies could hardly hold up the striped pyjamas that sagged from stooping shoulders to wooden clogs. Their ribs stuck out like picket fences in bodies so thin they seemed excessively tall.

The sickening smell of these remnants of humanity made handling them repulsive. We couldn't believe that even abnormal people could treat human beings this way. Scurvy and tuberculosis were rampant, and lice carried germs that caused secondary infections which produced open sores. Before handling them, we put DDT powder up our pant legs and down our shirtsleeves to protect us from the vermin. It was also mandatory for the general population at crossroads and bridges. Some of the servicemen got quite a kick out of spraying the powder down blouse fronts and up the skirts of the girls who had to pass the checkpoints.

In our mess tents we couldn't eat close to a wall opening, lest a clawing bony hand would snatch food from our mess tins. I'm afraid the German SS found no mercy on the part of our military after we discovered the death camps.

We had to streamline our admitting procedures in order to get them checked in as quickly as possible. Owen Swartz and I divided up one ward, with him on one side and myself on the other. While I was logging the admitting numbers from the slips, I gave him hell for going onto my side of the ward. He claimed he hadn't, and we saw where the confusion was coming from. The first two patients we admitted had the same name, except for one initial. There was one year's difference in age and they were from the same town in Russia. So we asked them in sign language if they knew each other. As soon as their eyes met from across the room, a transformation came over their beleaguered faces. It turned out they were brothers who had lost track of one another years before. Since they were both very seriously ill, they remained in bed on opposite sides of the ward. Later, once they regained their strength, they had a hell of a reunion.

One night, while everyone else slept, the guard at the front gate heard a squeaking noise. It was gradually getting louder. "Who goes there? Advance and be identified!" he bellowed. The noise kept approaching. Luckily, he didn't fire. Finally he was able to make out a Russian man pushing a wheelbarrow. In it was the Russian's pregnant wife. who was in labour. The poor soul was heading for a town in search of a doctor. The guard notified our medical officer on call and the woman gave birth to a daughter early that morning in our hospital. I remember the remarks around the unit—maternity was certainly a far cry from war surgery! Later that day, May 8, 1945, the war ended.

The nurses tried to talk the woman into naming the baby Victoria for VE Day, commemorating victory in Europe. As one might expect, a Russian name was given—which could have been Victoria, for all we knew.

For weeks we had been hearing rumours that the Germans had surrendered, so we didn't believe the first announcements that reached our unit. For some time we had been hearing the same phrase repeated by the captured Germans: "All is kaput."[3] We kept wondering why our unit was staying in Bassum. Why not on to Berlin? But at noon we saw the tables, covered with white bedsheets, being carried out into the sun. Then came tangible proof of victory—eggs, peaches, chicken, chocolates, cigarettes, cigars, and champagne—it had to be true. It was a glorious spring day and VE Day had arrived!

"We made it through this damn war and now we can see our folks again," swam through my mind. Some of the men were interested in joining the war in the Pacific; I wanted a chance to go home first.

But little fears crept in: After five years, what changes will I see at home? How will I fit in and what will I do? We realized that we were no longer carefree kids. We had traded in our younger years; we would be returning home as men. I never knew the years I had missed until much later, when I watched my own children grow up as teenagers. But on that sunny day in May, the Union Jack was fluttering at the head of our tables. This was the celebration we had been waiting for.

Our unit was chosen from among six Canadian hospitals as the Canadian Occupation Force Hospital in Germany as a battle honour. With the war over, we were moved into a completely modern German naval hospital with electric elevators and circuit breakers instead of fuse boxes. This was quite a switch after sleeping on the ground and looking at washed out canvas walls. Some of the "peacetime casualties" we soon had to look after were cases of venereal disease. With the troops going on leave en masse, we were getting thirty VD cases a day, in addition to the assorted cases of pneumonia, broken legs, automobile accidents, and so on.

Since we had followed the British when the other Canadian units went into Holland, our unit had gone the furthest into Germany toward Berlin of any other Canadian unit except a company of the Canadian Parachute Battalion.

Bob Hope was entertaining the troops in Bad Zwischenahn, Germany, and we filled a truck to go see the show. His jokes were certainly more ribald than the ones he told on television! Thousands of troops filled the stands, and we were looking right down onto Bob Hope's platform. He was cracking jokes and making remarks about the troops—he had a close bond with all of us. At the end everybody stood up clapping wildly to give him a standing ovation.

Time passed slowly. I was anxious to get home. Our hospital personnel were replaced one by one and I was posted to No. 5 Canadian Field Ambulance, RCAMC, a First Division unit stationed in Hilversum, Holland.

We were billeted onto an estate. Around us were fields that had come to life with acres upon acres of tulips, all in bloom. There was little to do except wait for a draft back to England. The Dutch girls, mostly blonde, were more than friendly. Quite a few moved into the barracks with the men, and love wasn't the only motivator. Some of them had lost their families during the invasion, while others were in need of food.

A group of eight Springhillers congregated one day and I snapped some photos. Wherever we were in the European theatre throughout the war, friends we had grown up with were always close by.

Finally we received word to break camp and soon we were back in England. I was posted to a draft of about two hundred men to return to Military Depot No. 6 in Halifax, Nova Scotia. I was appointed administrative clerk and was responsible for all the paperwork.

One of my responsibilities was to account for the missing clothing in our draft.[4] One day when I was anxious to go on leave with some of the other boys I left all the clothing books[5] in the barracks and locked the door behind me. When I got back, they were gone. Someone had been in to clean up and away they went. Captain Scott panicked, but I reminded him that if overseas soldiers lose their uniforms in battle, they get replaced free of charge. Along with the new books we were issued new clothes, and we were the best-dressed draft coming back to Canada.

I went on leave to Birmingham and Dunfermline to say goodbye to all my friends there. In my four and a half years overseas I had made so many friends it was impossible to see them all. But when I returned from leave ready to go home, there were no ships. I had to wait again. My next leave was to London, and I stopped dead in my tracks as the Palladium Theatre took me back in time. Block-long queues were waiting for the next showing of *Gone With the Wind*, which had been playing in 1941 when I first visited London. The more things change, the more they stay the same.

Finally we embarked from Southampton on the *Isle de France*, a huge ocean liner. Since we didn't have to dodge U-boats on the way back, the trip was only five days instead of the two weeks we spent in the *Andes*.

When we glided into Halifax Harbour, we could make out a large billboard on the breakwater of the yacht squadron in Point Pleasant Park: THE LAST DIAMOND UP SIGN. Canadian advances from the D-Day beaches to the front lines were guided by diamond up signs, and the way back to the rear was signalled by diamond down signs. We had followed the diamond up signs to the war's end, and now the last one brought us home. I really appreciated that welcoming. "This is Nova Scotia," I thought. "Thank God we're home."

NOTES

1. Luftwaffe: German Air Force.

2. White Brigade: Belgian underground.

3. "All is kaput": "Everything is finished."

4. This Canadian draft consisted of 250 servicemen.

5. Clothing books: Books that listed all the items of clothing that belonged to each serviceman.

6. Veteran, Student, Miner, and Doctor

WHEN I CLIMBED ONTO THE BUS AT THE HALIFAX DEPOT, FIVE SPRINGHILL VETS WERE RIGHT BEHIND ME. FINALLY WE ARRIVED at the bandstand at the bottom of Main Street, and I looked out at the crowds lining both sides of the street. I recognized many of them. We were led up to the bandstand one by one to the sound of honking cars, and introduced to the townspeople. Each of us was supposed to say a few words into the microphone, but Mayor A. J. Mason grabbed the microphone from the second soldier and abruptly ended the ceremonies. He must have gotten bored with all the pomp and circumstance. I was more interested in seeing my folks anyway, so being robbed of my two minutes in the sun was actually a relief.

One girl called me by name, and I hadn't the foggiest notion who she was. Finally I recognized Lorraine Corkum, my neighbour from two houses up the road. The last time I saw her she was twelve and now she was seventeen. Five years makes quite a difference at that age.

From the bandstand I could see my dad in his blue serge suit, white shirt, and tie, my stepmother in a subdued print dress, and my sister sporting a brightly coloured print dress partially hidden by a brown jacket. The only contact we had had for four and a half years was with paper and pen—there hadn't been so much as a phone call.

As I stepped off the bandstand, neighbours and friends streamed in to welcome me, and I made my way against the tide up to where my family stood. I grabbed hold of Dad's hand and we gave each other a mighty hug. We felt the happiness but didn't express too much outwardly, like the Scotsmen we are. I met my niece for the first time as my sister held her up two inches from my nose, and then Audrey put her arms around me for a heartfelt hello before turning me over to my stepmother. It was an emotional moment and thoughts flooded through me: "It's just so nice to be back," and "The army part of my life is nearly over." I still had to be discharged; technically this was just another leave—but the end was in sight.

With the war over, I decided to go to medical school. First of all, my tuition was paid with re-establishment credits. Single vets were entitled to sixty dollars a month for living expenses, while married fellows qualified for ninety dollars. I knew this wouldn't go too far paying rent in Halifax, buying food, and investing in medical books at twenty dollars each. But it was a start. Casualty handling had rubbed off on me; by this time I felt at home looking after the sick and injured. Dad had already asked a friend of his who was president of Acadia University about the pre-medical program there. But I wanted to go to Dalhousie, and so began to inquire. The colleges had already begun the school year in September, but Dalhousie would be starting a new class in January to accommodate us late arrivals from overseas. This saved us a year.

While waiting in No. 6 Depot for my final discharge from the army, I was able to finalize arrangements to attend Dalhousie in January 1946. Two hundred of us would be starting in mid-year, and would swell the ranks of the freshmen who had begun in the fall.

After four lonely Christmases overseas, this one was spent at home. It was a normal Canadian Christmas, with gifts, lots of food, and above all, no worries. During my time overseas, I had never been injured other than getting hit by the odd piece of shrapnel. But over the Christmas holidays I was chasing a rabbit and managed to drive a spruce tree branch into my knee joint. It hurt more than anything that had happened to me during the war! I was taken to our family doctor to have the piece of branch removed.

I went to Halifax the day after New Year's to sign up for college—five years to the day since I'd ridden the bus there to enlist.

At twenty-three, I was five years older than the freshmen. Needless to say, the sophomores didn't make us jump through the hoops of a freshman initiation. I got credit for the correspondence course I had taken while in England, but had to sweat it out in Latin class. Since I hadn't taken any Latin in high school, I had to complete the equivalent of a four-year course during my first six months at Dalhousie in addition to the regular first year courses. I studied a total of four hours a night, six nights a week, and it saw me through.

I took a room along with Bob Willett from Moncton on LeMarchant Street—one block from campus. My re-establishment credits amounted to one month in college for each month in the army. Since a college year was only eight months long, I had over seven years of college coming to me, as long as I made the grade each year. I also received sixty dollars a month to go towards living expenses. To this day, the army owes me four months, but I figure it all comes out in the wash.

The chemistry class included a lot of mathematics that the veterans had never been taught. The group that started in the fall had four months on us; we were just given sets of notes to study. Despite our handicap, everyone in the January to July class passed, whereas some of the first group failed. Sid Baxter, who later became a dentist, and I both scored one hundred per cent on our final papers. We had studied together, and had evidently concentrated on the right sections.

During my second summer I went home to work, and the mines were on strike. I got a job with the town and did everything from digging ditches to mowing the grass at the bandstand. One time I was helping to dig a sewer line and we hit solid rock. There were no pneumatic drills at that time, so we had to use a star drill and a maul to get through the rock. Not everyone was willing to put their hand in jeopardy by holding the drill while someone else swung at it with a twenty-pound maul. Joe Dembronski and I were a good team, and we worked away at the rock. When the holes were deep enough, the rock was blasted with dynamite. Some of the other workers who shied away from the star drill shovelled out the rock from where we had worked. Meanwhile, Joe and I moved over onto the next site. The ditch was about ten feet deep, and suddenly tons of rock and mud caved in from the side onto the men who had taken our places. The man with only his head sticking up suffered chest injuries, while the other fellow was able to scurry out.

I was on my way home that day wearing some awfully muddy clothes when I came upon Gordie Bigelow. He introduced me to his girlfriend, Helen Dewar. I'm afraid I couldn't have made much of a first impression on my future wife.

Meanwhile, having completed two years of pre-med, I was waiting to hear back from Dalhousie. Finally word came that I was accepted into medical school. There was only room for 58 qualified applicants out of 250, and we lost 6 after the first-year exams. Most were veterans, because we had received a ten per cent advantage over our classmates.

Well into the first term a law student friend came up to congratulate me on my scholarship. "What scholarship?" I asked, bewildered. They had posted it on the law bulletin board instead of the board in the medical school by mistake. The five hundred dollars was a godsend, since I had five more years of college ahead of me.

Major Tabbie Bethune kept track of the servicemen who had been discharged from No. 7 Canadian General Hospital. I typed up all the news about what the vets were doing in civilian life and we produced a newsletter called *Seven Sayings*, which was modelled after the unit newsletter we had printed overseas. We continued with this for a few years, sending them to all the unit personnel for whom we had addresses.

That summer I worked in the No. 1 coal seam with Jack Whitewood. Jack was a seasoned miner in his fifties who had fractured his leg in the mines, and was just now returning to work for the first time. Since he was not medically fit to work on the coal face,[1] Jack was assigned to the 5100 west level[2], which had not been used for some time. This was my first chance to work in the mines. I laced up the heavy boots with the steel toecaps, put on coveralls, a protective safety hat with a place to hold the lamp, a belt to hold the lamp battery, and last but not least, a pair of heavy leather gloves. My clothes were stiff and smelled like new, while all around me was the stale smell of dried sweat from pit clothes that had ridden the trolleys into the bowels of the earth more times than I could imagine. My spanking new lunch can and water can were full, and I recalled the old miners' superstition: if you empty your water can while still on the surface, you mustn't refill it to go in the mine that day. The next time I put those same pit clothes on, my face and hands would be streaked with coal dust even before leaving the washhouse.

The miners were all standing around, waiting for the man-rake.[3] The low trolleys were outfitted like stair steps where the men sat. On the way down that morning of my initiation, everyone was joking around or kidding one another in quiet conversation. There was no hint of danger. But I soon discovered it lurked in the back of everyone's mind.

As we left the early-morning light, stepped into the door of the bankhead, and took our seats on the trolley, I noticed a new smell. It was "the mine smell," not unpleasant but awfully distinctive. It was the odour of air that had been pumped down into the mine, circulating three miles through the maze of underground tunnels and mixing with the sweat of hundreds of toiling bodies. It was air that had combined with the rancid smell of exploding dynamite—used to loosen the coal—and the methane gas that had been trapped in the million-year-old solidified vegetation.

We descended into the pit as my headlamp shone a bright beam onto the blackness in front of me, while the other lamps cast lights and shadows across the trolley. All other light receded as we hurtled towards the depths. The temperature was in the seventies, and very constant. In some places the roof was quite low, supported by steel railroad rails which were in turn supported by wooden packs[4] on either side of the slopes.[5] Gaping hollows overhead showed where rock had broken loose and fallen onto the slope; in these sections, the roof was so high that my light was only a faint beam at the top. The trolley wheels clickety-clacked as someone broke into a song, their voice reverberating in the cavernous underground.

Jack and I got off at the 5100 west level. The company wanted to send timber down a tunnel to a wall[6] below, and so Jack and I were assigned to make room so that the four-foot-high boxes[7] of timber could pass through. Since there was no compressed air line on that level for running pneumatic drills, all our work had to be done by pick, axe, saw, wooden props, and a healthy ration of muscle power. He had me shovelling chipped stone, sawing poles, driving wedges, loading stone into the box, and cutting props.[8] Jack taught me a lot about mining that summer, including what to do when the loose rock you're shoring up overhead gives way.

One night I dropped into a bowling alley and came upon Helen Dewar and Gordie Bigelow's sister. Helen and Gordie had broken up by that time. We bowled a few games, and then I walked Helen home. We started keeping steady company, going to shows, bike rides, and so on. Since she was six years younger, we hadn't known each other while we were growing up, plus I had been overseas. When I came home after my first year of medicine, marriage was in the air.

We went to New Glasgow by train for our honeymoon, since I didn't have a car. Helen's sister's husband, who was a travelling salesman, came and picked us up at the hotel when the honeymoon was over and drove us back to Springhill.

Expenses would be much higher in Halifax for the two of us, so I worked as much overtime as I could that summer. One day I was working in another section of the mine with Henry Mackenzie, and we were told to move the pan.[9] It was too long, having been sent down to the No. 1 mine by mistake. We were told to take it down a newly undercut coal face.[10] The pan was about 150 pounds of steel—ten feet long and two feet wide. Henry was up front and on the downhill end while I was carrying the back end. He lost his footing. The front end of the pan slid along the base of the coal face and jammed where the coal had been undercut.

Henry could run downhill to get out of the way, but I could only back up. I said to myself, "If I drop it, it's going to crush my toes. I've got to lower it down." As I bent over, the coal face collapsed onto the pan. I was trying to dodge between the packs when the roof came down on me. I managed to get between the packs as chunks of rock were falling off my back. My back was scraped and my leg was trapped under the rubble. Looking down, I saw trickles of dust, which meant there was more to come. I figured a broken leg is better than a totally crushed one. So I gave it a big yank and luckily pulled it free. I huddled in between the packs just before more of the roof let go. When I got home, I told Helen I'd slid on my back going down the slope, and she never did find out what happened until years later.

After a couple of months in the mine, it was time to hit the books again. Helen and I moved into a ramshackle building on Bland Street in Halifax that had been reserved for us by friends who were living on the ground floor. As I parked the half-ton truck carrying all of our worldly possessions, the first thing I noticed was that the front steps seemed to come out as far as the sidewalk, and that the front door faced the grain elevators. Helen, my stepmother, and I cautiously walked up to the front door, and the wood siding, which had given up most of its paint, gave me a depressing foretaste of what was to come. From the dingy front corridor, we went upstairs to our rooms on the second floor. Before we even got there, Helen and I were somber.

The look on Helen's face as she gazed blankly across the dark, scrawny rooms was a story in itself. My stepmother later remarked that if she had had a camera to take Helen's picture at that moment, her fortune would have been made. The bare light bulbs begged for fixtures. The only furnishings, if you could call them that, were wall calendars—one outdated and the other pinned behind the door to hide the official rental policy. This turned out to be intentional on the landlord's part because we later discovered he was charging more than the legal limit. All the windows looked onto buildings no more than six feet away.

Our clothes closet was a wooden shelf hidden by a curtain in the so-called living room. We certainly wondered about the judgment of our friends. Like many things in life, we learned to live with it since we were stuck.

One day Helen baked a lovely lemon meringue pie. She had set it on the table to cool, and asked me to go out and pick up some bread. Our coat hook was over the kitchen table, and as I reached for my coat, you can guess what happened. That's right, it cleaned off the meringue. It must have been hard for her in those early days, especially since I was at school all day and had to study 'til eleven o'clock at night.

This second year of medicine was particularly tough because the college had shortened several of the courses from two years to a year and a half. This meant we had to complete all of the second-year material in half a year. Come Christmastime we wrote four finals, and if we missed two we were out for the year, if not for good.

At the end of the school year we immediately put our furniture in storage and went back to Springhill. The manager of Dominion Steel & Coal Corp. Ltd. (DOSCO) had approached Dad earlier asking, if I wanted to work in the mines that summer. I was glad to be working in the mines again; that summer the job was in No. 4 mine, mostly at the 7100 wall.

During the miners' two-week vacation I was given a job at the pumps, so I worked straight through. The air pumps cleared water out of the mine so it wouldn't flood. I was to watch the pump transferring water from the lower level to the upper level. From below, it was pumped into a box at my level that was about four feet by four feet. Then I pumped it up, and eventually it went out to the mine pond. I had to make sure the water level in the box didn't get so low that the pump started sucking air, or so high that it would overflow. So I fashioned a little boat, ran a wire through the top, and attached a flag to the wire. By floating this boat in the box, I could monitor the pumping by sitting back on the far side of the slope. For the two weeks I was on that pump I was able to study Cunningham's *Anatomy of the Forearm*, which I brought in with me each day, protected by an oilcloth cover.

If you've heard stories of rats in the mines, they're true: I got to know five of them almost by name. Each noon hour as I unpacked my sandwiches, I could hear the loose coal or stone rustling. Since it was pitch black, except where the light on my forehead was pointing, I couldn't see them until I pointed in their direction. There they were, six or seven feet away, grey and about ten inches long. One had a crooked tail and another had a cut ear; I could tell them apart. Some would scurry away and hide, while others just stood there fixing their beady eyes on me. They knew I was about to eat, and they were even hungrier than usual because all the other men were on holiday. Miners' fingers were always black, so we would eat down to one corner of the sandwich, and throw the blackened bit away. This had become, quite literally, the rats' bread and butter. They anxiously waited for this inevitable morsel. It was like a dog that knows when the paper boy's due; at 7:05 he waits, without fail.

That summer I worked just about every job in No. 4 mine: duffing[11] on the coal face, building stone walls to protect the roof, operating a tugger engine,[12] working on the conveyor line, drawing packs,[13] and moving timber. One time as I was putting timber on the pan, the mine bumped. This was the first time I was underground during a bump, which is a release of pressure in the stratification of rock and coal as a result of mining. A surge of air swept up the wall and brought coal dust along with it; it was about ten minutes before I could see. No one was hurt, and we continued working.

Generally the miners were happy after small bumps like that, because they relieved the pressure from the roof and often loosened up the coal face. This made for an easy shift, shovelling coal from the face to the pan line.

But these small bumps could still be dangerous. One day, just after a contract miner left his spot at the coal face, the mine bumped and the face let go into about a six-foot pile of coal right where he had been working.

The men were motherly to me. "Be sure you wear your gloves, Arnold," they'd say. "You're going to be a doctor one day and you'll need good hands." That summer I had occasion to walk up the auxiliary slope[14] when the trolley was out of order. Familiarity with this slope came in handy quite a few years later.

Back in Halifax for my third year in medical school, we found much more civilized lodgings. The residence of Mr. and Mrs. William Bradley in the Hydrostone area was immaculately clean, airy, and full of light. Our suite included a large sitting room, and I was later given my own study when an elderly gentleman moved out. There were apple trees in back, a lawn all around, and the neighbouring buildings didn't crowd us. It was the opposite of our rooms on Bland Street.

At the end of the school year, we decided to stay in Halifax so as not to give up our wonderful set of rooms. I took a job at the Victoria General Hospital as an orderly, for which I was certainly well qualified. I soon wound up on the neurosurgical unit, which was the only such unit east of Montreal at that time. I very much appreciated the opportunity to work on this highly specialized unit, where brain surgeries were not uncommon.

One man of about thirty had received a traumatic frontal lobotomy on a construction job—a rock from a construction explosion had removed his forehead and part of his brain. One consequence of this type of injury is loss of inhibitions. One afternoon he was telling the ward patients and nurses he was going to get married. A young blonde nurse turned to him and asked, "Why?"

He immediately answered: "So I can have it any time I want it." The nurse found a reason to leave the ward in a hurry.

Before I knew it, my clinical clerkship had arrived: the fourth year of medical school. Most of our time was spent in the wards, doing histories and attending patients. For instance, one month we had to attend every maternity at the Grace Maternity Hospital, while still being responsible for the material presented in all our lectures.

That year I bought my first car—a dark blue 1937 Plymouth. Since it took me a while to learn to drive and get a permit, I kept riding my bicycle from our North End home to the hospital in the South End, with the car parked in the driveway. The only time I had ever driven was over in Marston Green, England. We had been burning coke in the main furnace for the hospital and the supply had run low. So I went out back and hopped in the three-ton truck that had been parked too far away from the coke pile. I proceeded to back up, my foot slipped off the clutch, and the truck went so far into the pile that we didn't have to pick up the shovel.

This Plymouth wasn't in tip-top shape. Fuses were always shorting out and the cooling system was half–plugged up with sludge. I ended up learning about second-hand cars as fast as I was learning about surgery.

One day a "heart attack patient" was admitted to the ward. He was a man of about fifty, and by the way he was breathing, I felt he had a lung problem instead. It sounded like pleurisy to me. I mentioned this to the chief, and it was a nice feeling when the diagnosis was corrected to pleurisy. Another time I was examining a World War One veteran of about sixty who had been admitted to Camp Hill Hospital on numerous occasions for "congestive heart failure." I noted the lack of congestion at the base of the lungs, which didn't fit with the diagnosis. On my way out, I mentioned this to Dr. Steeves, who was in charge of the department, and suggested thyroid function tests. About a week later, Dr. Steeves stopped me in the hall to say that the fellow's low thyroid had been causing his recurring heart failure.

After the fourth year, we went directly into internship without a summer vacation. We had passed the written exams, including the Dominion Council exams, which permitted us to practice anywhere in Canada, with reciprocity in the British Empire, as well as some parts of the United States. With the title of "doctor," we could still only practice as an intern under the supervision of a doctor. I felt a bit like a young bird with wings that couldn't quite fly.

I chose the hospital in Charlottetown, Prince Edward Island, for part of my internship because four medical officers I knew from overseas were working there. It was a strange hospital in a strange city, but when I heard that Dr. Gordie Lea told Tabbie Bethune that he'd look after me like a father, I took comfort. Gordie had been a major and was now a chest specialist at the hospital in PEI. The other veterans from No. 7 Canadian General Hospital were Major Gilbert Houston, an ear, nose, and throat specialist; Major Hal Shaw, a pathologist; and Lieutenant Colonel Don Campbell, a surgeon.

I moved into a room on the hospital's first floor and was on call twenty-four hours a day for obstetrics and whatever else came up. As well, I was to learn anaesthetics and otolaryngology,[15] assist at surgery, write up case histories, and be generally available.

Dr. Kent Irwin trained me in obstetrics and gynecology. He was a very friendly man of medium height. After about two weeks in the hospital, I was called for one of his deliveries, so was scrubbed and went in to check on the mother. Meanwhile, Dr. Irwin, who lived about twenty minutes from the hospital, had taken the call but was delayed. The woman, who was about thirty-two, turned out to be a personal friend of his. She was lying on the table with a sheet over her, staring at the ceiling, which was a good thing because that way she couldn't see my face when I checked on the position of the baby. I reached in and felt the cord. It was crushed between the head and the vaginal wall. Since the only oxygen a baby receives is through the cord, it could have died or become brain damaged in a matter of minutes. I was wildly signalling to the nurses from my hidden spot down below. I couldn't wait for Dr. Irwin; something had to be done right away.

My heart was beating wildly as I reached for the forceps for the first time. I was thinking, "If I don't get this baby out alive, this could be the end of my medical career, because I'm doing something I'm not allowed to do." But I had absolutely no choice. The nurse frantically phoned Dr. Irwin, but I managed to get the baby out some time before he arrived. Fortune smiled on the baby—and me—that day, and it certainly helped boost my rapport with the doctors.

My face was sure red one day when I learned how patients try to fool doctors. A woman was admitted with "arthritis of the back" and so I proceeded to take her history and do the physical exam. She kept pulling the bedclothes about her, and in the middle of the exam I was called away to the emergency room. When I came back I began examining the left side of the chest. "You've already done that breast," she said curtly. So I examined the right side and then ordered an X-ray of the lower spine. The next day, Dr. Lea nabbed me on my way out of the operating room. "Did you actually examine that patient?" he asked wide-eyed.

"Yes."

"Did you see the X-ray?"

"No."

He brought me to the X-ray department and pointed to a lesion on the spine that was obviously a metastatic cancer. She had hidden from me the large cancer of the left breast when she instructed me to examine the right side for the second time. She just didn't want me to find that cancer. When she admitted to Dr. Lea she had fooled, me I wasn't any less embarrassed.

After ten weeks in Charlottetown, I left to continue my internship in Halifax. I had no idea at that point that I would begin my medical practice on the Island the following year.

My internship was in several services of the Victoria General Hospital and the Children's Hospital: ambulance, urology, surgical, gynecology, medical, pediatrics, and neurosurgery. I continued to do examinations, write histories, make diagnoses, and start treatment. Of every forty-eight hours, I had twelve hours off in which I could get sleep, if nothing else happened. For all this, I received the magnificent sum of one hundred dollars a year, or eight dollars and thirty-three cents a month. Even with uniforms, laundry, and meals provided, it was tough to support a wife on this! My earnings from the mines in the summer, and the balance of the savings bond that had been taken out when I was overseas, provided just enough for essentials.

Whenever an ambulance went to pick up a patient who weighed over two hundred pounds and lived on the fourth or fifth floor of a house, I was the ambulance orderly—or so it seemed. One call took us to a mission on the outskirts of Halifax during a major snowstorm. A stone wall surrounded the estate and the driveway was impenetrable. The driver and I had to drag the heart attack victim over snowbanks on a wood-and-canvas stretcher, and the drifts were high. After labouring through snow up to our armpits, we got him to the ambulance. The man was having severe chest pains, his skin was sweaty and his face pale. I gave him oxygen in the ambulance and we delivered him to the emergency room of the Victoria General.

One day while I was on Dr. Vic Mader's surgical service (as Colonel Mader he had taken our unit into France) he operated on Dr. Harold Simpson, my family doctor and the senior doctor of the Springhill Medical Clinic. Dr. Simpson had cancer of the left lung. While I was being scrubbed for the operation, I overheard Dr. Mader's conversation with the other doctors. All of the cancer could not be removed. Coincidentally, I was on a medical service about a month later when Dr. Simpson returned to the hospital and suddenly went into auricular fibrillation. I attended to him that night, immediately putting him under sedation and using oxygen and digitalis.[16] His heartbeat became regular within a half-hour of treatment. He and I had always been quite close; I had known him my whole life. He had removed that one-and-a-half-inch-long tree branch from my knee that first summer I was home from the war.

In the Children's Hospital, our diagnosis of cystic fibrosis was rather primitive by today's standards. We would scrape the child's feces from a diaper and make multiple dilutions of it. Then we would take a control feces, dilute it, and put them both on undeveloped X-ray plates. We'd leave it sit a day, and then wash it off. If the patient had cystic fibrosis, the feces would lack the digestive enzymes necessary to digest the film from the plates. It was a stinky but effective test. Nowadays, a sweat test from a palm or footprint is all that is needed.

On May 16, 1952, I graduated as an intern and received my degrees: MD (Medical Doctor), CM (Master of Surgery), and LMCC (Licentiate of the Medical Council of Canada). This last degree allowed me to practice medicine anywhere in the British

Empire, and with reciprocity in some states of the United States. At the ceremony I was sitting next to Angus Swansberg, who had been an orderly with me overseas, and two parcels were passed over to us. They were custom-engraved desk clocks from Dr. Tabbie Bethune, our army major. Mine reads "To RAB from CMB 16th of May 1952." This special recognition from Tabbie was very touching.

NOTES

1. Coal face: The working surface where the coal is mined.

2. 5100 west level: A level is a passageway from the slope into which the coal is mined. This level was 5,100 feet below the surface, and the walkway was on a thirty-degree slope.

3. Man-rake: A trolley that carries men into the mine.

4. Packs: Hardwood timber used to support the roof.

5. Slope: Passageway that provides access from the surface to the levels.

6. Wall: Working area between the two levels where the coal is mined.

7. Boxes: Trollies.

8. Props: Timber that holds up the beam that supports the roof.

9. Pan: Miners throw coal onto the pan, a large steel trough, which carries the coal to the trollies.

10. Undercut coal face: Machines with a three-inch cutter bar cut the base of the coal face to a depth of six feet. This enables the miners to mine the coal more easily.

11. Duffing: After the coal is cut, this is the process of removing the fine coal before repositioning the pan line close to the newly undercut coal face.

12. Tugger engine: A hydraulic engine, run by compressed air, for pulling equipment such as a trolly or a scoop run.

13. Drawing packs: Taking the packs out so the roof can fall in.

14. Auxiliary slope: A slope providing an alternate route back to the surface.

15. Otolaryngology: Ear, nose, and throat treatment.

16. Digitalis: A drug used to strengthen the heart.

7. Reviving a Dead Man and the Interminable Maternity

WITH THE "BIG DAY," THE GRADUATION BALL, AND THE FANFARE BEHIND ME, I WAS ANXIOUS TO PRACTICE MEDICINE AND SURGERY on my own—and to get paid for it. But I would soon become privy to a trade secret: collecting money wasn't so easy in the days before medicare.

The first of the year—before completing my internship—I had called the Springhill Medical Centre to see if they would have a place for me. They said, "We have all the doctors we need." After what I knew about Dr. Simpson, I couldn't very well have said, "Well, you'll be needing one before long." In any case, I received an invitation to practice there just before graduation, but I had already committed myself to take over a practice in Prince Edward Island by that time. The date was set for July, which allowed me some time for a vacation. But the Springhill Medical Centre was unflagging. They made me an offer I couldn't refuse: five hundred dollars a month for May and June, so I cast my vacation to the wind and started in Springhill the day after graduation.

My first call was to see a nine-year-old girl who had badly burned the bottoms and tops of her feet. She lived in the "Rows," a residential section of town the coal company had built for miners around the turn of the century. This girl had wandered over to the town dump in her bare feet and stepped onto burning underground debris. Her feet were covered with dirt from the dump, so I cleansed them, gave her a sulfa drug to stop the germs from multiplying, bandaged her feet, and followed up with daily visits.

As I recalled from childhood, the mine "check-off" was a system that allowed the miners to buy family medical coverage for fifty cents a week. The pre-paid medical plan was ahead of its time, except in one respect: if the miner was out of work due to injury, his family was still entitled to free medical care even though he was no longer paying in. The doctor wouldn't get paid until the man was back on the job. The miners were ahead of the game, while the doctors were behind the eight ball. The check-off continued until well after the 1958 disaster, at which point it was replaced by Maritime Medical Care and other plans.

I worked with four doctors at the medical centre, and we were busy from eight in the morning until ten or eleven at night, six days a week. We started the day with surgery, then looked after in-patients and out-patient emergencies. We each made several house calls before supper, and then kept office hours in the evening. Surgery was frequently necessary due to the injuries in the mines. There were crushed limbs and broken backs from roofs caving in, many broken bones, and miscellaneous cuts, bruises, and tears. It seemed like we did more orthopaedic surgery than the doctors at the Victoria General Hospital. Our surgical repertoire included abdominal, orthopaedic, skin grafts, amputations, hysterectomies, and splenectomies.[1] The only surgeries we sent elsewhere were the brain and lung surgical cases.

During my first week, I got an emergency call from Miller Corner in Springhill. A panicked voice on the other end of the phone said, "I think Grandpa died," gave me an address, and hung up. It was mid-afternoon. I grabbed my emergency case and hurried out to the house on the west side of town. In the kitchen, an old white-haired gentleman was slumped down in a rocking chair. His head was slung forward. I examined him; he wasn't breathing, there was no heartbeat, his pupils were dilated, and his face had a bluish cast. Medically speaking, he was dead. There must have been half a dozen family members gathered round, staring intently. Some were sobbing, while others just stood there in shock.

"I'm just a new doctor here," I thought. "I'm not prepared to see people die in the home. Nobody taught me what to do about this."

In my emergency kit was an assortment of medical ampoules.[2] I grabbed some adrenaline, filled a syringe, and plunged the needle directly into the man's heart muscle. I had to go straight to the heart, since blood had stopped circulating. I pulled the needle out and stepped back. The old man opened his eyes, raised up his head, and said, "What happened?"

Well, I can't describe the transformation on the faces around me. This was a miracle! They had been watching me inject the adrenaline, expecting me to say, "Well, he's dead." Instead, his heart started back up again. The teary eyes were suddenly lit up with an indescribable joy. And the ninety-year-old was talking as if nothing had happened.

I said, "Well, you had a spell. Apparently you're a lot better now. How do you feel?"

He said, "I feel all right." I told him to get plenty of rest and bid them all goodbye.

The gentleman lived several more weeks. That family must have spread the news, because from then on I got most of the calls from Miller Corner. Now, I may have seemed like Harry

Houdini to the family, but this was an accepted procedure for advanced cardiac life support. Nowadays, modern equipment is used to defibrillate someone with a cardiac arrest, and there are newer drugs to maintain the heartbeat.

At that time, the cobalt bomb was the newest cancer treatment, and a hospital in London, Ontario, had the only technology in the world. Arrangements were made for Dr. Simpson to go for treatments, and he asked me to come along to look after the oxygen tanks and so on. We took the train, and he was in the bottom sleeper bed while I was right above him. I tied my bathrobe belt to my wrist and let the other end of the belt hang down so he could wake me if need be. He could hardly breathe during the trip, and I was relieved once we arrived in London.

The doctors at the London Hospital showed me the equipment and techniques used for the cobalt bomb radiation treatment. Each lung cancer patient, for example, was fitted with a plaster cast. The cast was then cut, and ties were attached so that it could be reused for each treatment. Ports were marked on the plaster so that the cobalt bomb rays would criss-cross under the ports, centering on the cancerous area in the patient's body. This way, the cancer got the highest intensity of radiation.

As I was listening to this explanation, a voice came across the loudspeaker to evacuate the room because a patient was due for treatment. I turned towards the door and a beautiful woman was coming towards me in a wheelchair. Her hair was covered by a turban. I looked into her pale face as she wheeled past. Her expression was blank, and I felt a vague glimmer of recognition. Only later was I able to put the jigsaw puzzle together, with the help of one of the doctors. The Argentinian beauty, Eva Peron, had come to North America to treat her cancer. And I had seen her face on postage stamps ever since my early days as a collector, beginning in the eighth grade.

When my two months were up at the medical centre, Helen and I took off for Prince Edward Island. We were a thousand dollars richer, and I was far richer in medical experience. Some months before, the doctors in Charlottetown had told me that the village of St. Peter's Bay needed a doctor, so we settled into a bungalow on the northeast shore of the Island in this village of about two hundred families. The nearest hospital was seventeen miles away, and I was in for my share of surprises.

Our house looked right out onto the bay and further north, onto the peninsula. I could throw stones from the front lawn into the bay. Our house stood facing north, then came the lawn, the road, the railroad tracks, and the water. St. Peter's Bay was a sleepy little village, until someone got into a fight. The north side fought with the south side. This seemed to be the tradition, and there was very little likelihood it would change. When it was time to build a school, they couldn't agree where to put it. So schools were built on both sides of the bay. To me, an outsider, this seemed ludicrous considering the total number of children. To the locals it was as natural as could be. You see, the Catholic church was on the north side and the Protestant church was on the south side....

Seventeen miles to the east was Souris (pronounced "Souree"), thirty-five miles to the west was Charlottetown, and seventeen miles to the south was Montague. Potato farms surrounded the village. The fishing villages that dotted the coast east of St. Peter's Bay were populated by lobstermen and tuna fishermen and their families.

I served a total population of four to five thousand people scattered among these villages. I had hospital privileges in the two large hospitals in Charlottetown, as well as in Souris and Montague. I was also given the coroner's appointment for Kings and Queens Counties, which accounted for two-thirds of the

Island. My rates were certainly modest: three dollars for an office visit and thirty-five dollars for total maternity care.

With no drug stores for seventeen miles, I had to take their place and dispense medicines. If an office call came to five dollars, including medicine, and I only took in two or three dollars cash (which wasn't uncommon). I was either providing free medical care or giving away medicine I had already paid for. Along with the actual medicines, I had to buy the boxes, labels, and bottles to put them in. Taking the place of a drug store was a losing proposition, but I had no choice. All I could do was hope for payment later during lobster season or at potato harvest time.

Just a few houses down the road from us lived Dr. Roddie MacDonald, an old Scots gentleman of about ninety-six who was still practicing medicine. He only saw a handful of patients whom he had been looking after for years. Dr. Roddie was always immaculately dressed; his fine white hair was predictably combed back with each hair in its place. Each birthday I would take out the Drambuie, go to his home, and toast his health with him. This became a ritual. On one such occasion, which must have been his hundredth birthday, the news reporters descended and swarmed him with questions. Finally Dr. Roddie got peeved and announced: "I've lived so long because I eat porridge." The following day's newspapers carried the story nationwide!

When Dr. Roddie helped in the inoculation clinics in the schools, he used to get riled at the younger nurses who always tried to carry his medical case or supplies. He'd say: "The younger generation just won't let a person be a gentleman." And when the Queen came to Charlottetown, Dr. Roddie was introduced to her as the oldest practicing doctor in the British Empire. She smiled when he said: "I didn't know why God has let me live so long, but now I know why."

Later, when Dr. Roddie was made a knight of St. Gregory, the highest honour the Catholic Church can bestow on a layman, I attended the service. Still delivering babies at ninety-six, he was an amazing individual. And he continued to drive his own car—with a heavy foot on the accelerator.

One day while I was having lunch, the phone rang. A frantic mother was on the line. "Little Johnnie swallowed a dime! What will I do? What will I do?"

Without thinking twice I replied, "Put the dimes on a higher shelf." It's a wonder I ever built up a practice. But she calmed down and even laughed, and I told her the dime would go through with no problem. "And if you want the dime back, keep an eye on his bowel movements."

I was driving a 1938 Dodge that I had bought while interning. In preparation for winter, I put on "knobby" tires that had big round bumps and ridges on them. The muddy roads in spring and fall made travel difficult enough, but when they froze, foot-and-a-half-deep ruts formed. Anyone with tubeless tires was out of luck, because the ruts would batter the sidewalk, loosen the rims, and flatten the tires.

In the spring, I was attempting to negotiate my way through the mud to get to a patient six miles away who had had a stroke. I was ok on the level, but when I tried to take the car up a steep hill, it tried a shortcut straight through the hill. The front end never lifted and plowed right into the mud. When I backed up, I could see the imprint of the front bumper, headlights, and grill in the soft mud of the road. I had to wait until five o'clock the next morning, after the mud had frozen and before it had a chance to thaw. The patient was in partial paralysis by the time I got there, but I was able to bring his blood pressure down with medication, and this brought him some relief.

There were lots of rivers and ponds with sea trout in them one day and not the next, depending on their travels up and down the river. I always carried my fishing gear in the trunk, and on the way home from a house call I would often catch a half-dozen trout, averaging about a pound each. I made my own flies, so I carried all the necessary components: peacock hurl,[3] squirrel tail, deer hair, wool, feathers, silk, fur, silver foil, and of course, fish hooks. I could never predict where the trout would be. There might be beautiful deep holes in a river without a raise to a fly, but then I'd find trout in a foot-wide muskrat channel in a swamp, two to three feet deep. Once I was trying to keep the flies from getting tangled in the trees and they accidentally dropped into a shallow pool that looked about six inches deep. The line took off, and I lifted two trout out of there, about a pound apiece. Usually by the time winter came we had enough trout in the freezer to last until spring.

We were lucky the first winter, but every other year on the Island it snowed heavily. In January 1953, our first child, William George, was born. Dr. Kent Irwin delivered him at six pounds, twelve and a half ounces in one of the Charlottetown hospitals, and I was suddenly a proud father.

Between the wild duck, geese, and rabbits on the Island and the deer and moose I brought back from Nova Scotia in the fall, we managed to keep our freezer well stocked. Our neighbour Ralph Sanderson butchered his own cattle and sold T-bone, sirloin, and round steaks in his store, all for fifty-three cents a pound.

Money was scarce, and I soon discovered the doctor's role as banker. Many of my customers were indebted to me by wintertime, and I knew that the lobster fishermen who had large numbers of traps made more money in a month or two than I would make the whole year. It hurt when I saw some of them on my list of overdue accounts. But round about May 1, the beginning of lobster season, they'd start showing up at my door to settle their accounts. The first week, they would visit the banks to pay off their boat repairs, rope, and other gear expenses; by the second week, it was time to square the medical bills.

"How much interest do I owe?" one stocky fellow in a plaid lumberjack asked one day.

"None."

"Do you like lobsters?"

"You bet."

He smiled and took off. That was the end of that conversation. One evening, while I was examining a patient in my office, the doorbell rang, and rang, and rang. I couldn't for the life of me figure why they wouldn't just come in and sit down in the waiting room. I had to excuse myself to find out what was up. There, on the front step, was the fisherman, dressed in his rough fishing clothes.

"Got some lobsters for you, Doctor," he said offhandedly.

"Why thank you, Ross. Why don't you put them in the kitchen?"

"No, Doctor, think I'll leave them on the back step." I went around to the back door, and there was a large, wooden-slatted lobster crate, dripping and trailing strands of seaweed. It was about a hundred pounds of small live lobsters! No wonder he refused to put them in the kitchen. Helen and I stayed up a good part of the night cooking lobsters, and most of them went into the freezer. That year the frozen lobsters tasted wonderful; the next year we tried the same thing and they tasted like sawdust.

A veterinarian by the name of Stan Terceira, his wife Lily, and their son Robert moved in next door. We became good friends; we visited back and forth every day and our sons played together.

Stan had a simple sign by his front door: Dr. Terceira, DVM. One evening he heard a horse and cart pull into the yard. Parting the drapes, he saw a man tying the horse to a fence post. Soon a couple appeared at the door.

"Are you the doctor?" the young fellow asked.

"Yes, please come in."

Once seated, the man launched in: "She's not doin' well." His wife just sat there and listened.

Stan asked, "Is there good clean straw for the bed?" The young man fidgeted a bit, and nodded. "Is she off her feed?"

This time he exchanged puzzled looks with his wife, and bobbed his head.

"And when was she serviced?"

The man got up, clutched his hat awkwardly, and spit out, "Are you a medical doctor?"

Stan replied, "I'm a veterinarian," his face broke into a grin, and then he lost control. All along Stan had been picturing a cow, while the fellow was talking about his wife beside him who was having a miscarriage! Stan picked up the phone to tell me he was sending them over, and he could hardly talk for laughing.

After that, I got back at him when Lily was pregnant. My parting remarks to him at night were: "If you use the calving chains, be sure to throw a bucket of hot water on them in case I need them for Lily."

So then, naturally, Helen told Lily what to do to get even with me. Just after the baby is born she should let on that she's asleep, lying there on the table, and then suddenly kick me in the face. A few weeks later, Lily and I headed to Souris Hospital. Lily was having contractions, and I couldn't interest her in the lupines blooming by the roadside. When we reached the hospital, she was moved onto the bed by the obstetrical table, but she never made it to the table. I cut the cord, and the baby was set at the foot of the bed. Lily was partly under anaesthetic, and as I examined her, she drew back one foot and kicked. She didn't come near me, but damn near kicked the baby off the bed. The baby ended up wrapped around a rung at the foot of the bed. Later I told her she should be prosecuted for attempted infanticide, with Helen an accessory before the fact.

I was elected to the executive of the Medical Society of PEI and appointed to serve on the Maternal Health and Child Welfare Commission for the provincial government as well. Then I became a member of the Laboratory Council of the Island. This group, which relied on federally funded grants, was responsible for all laboratory services on the Island. Also at that time, the College of Family Practice of Canada was organized, and I soon became a charter member. I remained a member for twenty-five years, but became disillusioned when I saw it become more interested in empire building than in fostering post-graduate study, which was its mandate.

A call came in from a distraught husband. His wife was about to have her twelfth baby, and he pleaded with me to come immediately. This was a woman I had never seen before, and the family lived about eighteen miles away. I knew the farmhouse would be about six miles from the nearest telephone. Even though I had three maternity cases who could go into labour at any time, I had to go. As I drove up to the home, both the house and the barn looked terribly run down: shutters in disrepair and the siding riddled with peeling paint.

I went in and examined the woman. She looked about eighty, but her husband said she was forty-five. I could see the baby's head of hair, but the cervix wasn't fully dilated and the contractions stopped. The muscles of her womb seemed worn out. She was suffering from malnutrition and looked like a pencil with the eraser in the middle. The family was destitute. The kids were everywhere, and with very little furniture in the house, I had no choice but to wait in the car.

Every now and again someone would bolt out the door and yell at me to come in. But each time I examined her it was the same story; the contractions quit. The farmer served me humble fare at mealtimes. I began to feel like I was caught in a vise: I couldn't very well leave, but I had responsibilities to my other maternity cases. And nobody could reach me by phone! Soon I grew cold and uncomfortable as night fell, but I made the best of it in my car and managed to doze off a few times during the night.

I kept checking the baby's heartbeat with a fetoscope, and the fetal heart was normal. None of the textbooks in college mentioned this condition. Since the hospital cost money, the couple was quite unwilling to go.

After *thirty-six hours*, I finally announced that she was not ready to give birth, that I was leaving, and they were welcome to call me again. Sure enough, the farmer called a week later. I went back out to find the same condition, only this time I increased the dosage of pitocin. When intravenous didn't work, in desperation I injected a cc directly into the cervix. This only activated the cervix for two contractions, so I packed up my medical case and said goodbye once again. This time I was firm:

"She must go to the hospital. I will attend her there."

Two days later I got a call from the hospital in Souris. Either she or her husband must have gotten tired of the whole affair, because when she arrived at the hospital, she wasn't even having contractions. The hospital said they couldn't keep her until she was in labour. I advised the husband to take her back to the farm and wait it out. By this time, he must have been tearing his hair out: looking after his wife, trying to keep the twelve children in line, and trying to keep up with his farm work.

At the end of the second week she was back in the hospital—this time with contractions. I went, and although it looked more promising, it was still risky obstetrics. I still had to give her pitocin intravenously and, lo and behold, the cervix opened and I delivered a six-pound baby with low forceps. It was an easy delivery because the baby had been pushed down so far and for so long. It had been in the outlet position for two weeks, but it was healthy even though its nourishment had been minimal.

That was the last "planned" home delivery. From that point on, I notified my pre-natal patients that they would be delivered in the hospital, excepting emergencies.

One woman who knew I was no longer doing home deliveries decided to pull a fast one. She called me to her home, and once I got there, told me she had no intention of going to hospital. A woman was there to help, and she had multiple layers of newspapers sewn together to protect the bed. I examined her and found that there was plenty of time to go to hospital. Early in the pregnancy I had told her I only did hospital deliveries, except in emergency cases.

She said, "I'm having the baby at home no matter what you told me."

"I'll be in my car for fifteen minutes. If you join me, I'll take you to hospital. If not, I'll consider that you've dismissed me from your case." Sure enough, fifteen minutes later she stepped into the car. But that was only a short-term victory; she won in the end by stiffing me on the bill.

In the winter, emergency deliveries weren't all that uncommon during heavy snowstorms. Quite often doctors at the Charlottetown hospitals would ask me to look after patients who had planned their deliveries in Charlottetown. Typically, the husband or neighbour would come by driving horse and sleigh. Charging hooves and flying clumps of ice and snow added zest to the normal routine of house calls. I'd have to dodge the chunks of snow the horse kicked behind. Then, with the emergency over and the first horse tired out, there was usually a change of pace on the way back. The husband would hitch up an old plow horse, which made for a slow-motion ride back, two or three times longer than the trip in.

On other calls I made in a sled, I'd hunker down in my flight suit and full winter gear and the driver would throw a buffalo robe over me. I'd be set for an exciting sub-zero ride. I found the sound of the sled runners on the hard-packed snow quite soothing, and often dropped off to sleep during the five- or ten-mile trip.

The farmers knew the "winter roads" like their own palms. Sometimes they'd start out on a road and go through a farmyard, across an orchard, and into an open field, and then ride alongside the woods before pulling up to the farmhouse.

In the summertime we attended the church suppers in the area, so the ones in the Catholic church hall were no exception. The church and its high steeple dominated the far side of the bay. But the hall, directly across the road from the church, possessed no distinguishing features. One particular day when Bill was only a few months old, Helen and I walked in carrying the bassinet. The tables were set up for supper, and we were walking down the main aisle. I was headed for the back of the room so I could set Bill down before Helen and I went to supper. I was speaking with a lady I knew from the village, and apparently hadn't heard Mrs. McDonald talking to me from behind. After I deposited Bill in back and headed towards the centre of the room, Mrs. McDonald remarked loudly, so everyone could hear: "Oh, doctor, you didn't recognize your patient who was in hospital."

This sort of peeved me. She was putting me on the spot to her own advantage. I replied, "Oh, I'm sorry. I didn't recognize you with your clothes on."

Although Helen was ready to clobber me, I looked around and most everyone was grinning, except you-know-who. I didn't hear a peep out of her the rest of the night.

On weekends we took off in the car, exploring the areas around St. Peter's Bay. The area had been laid out in squares with surrounding roads by Lord Selkirk years ago, so self-navigation was easy with the help of a map. One sunny day, up on the north side of Greenwich, we left the end of the road, drove through a farmyard and some fields, and came to the sand dunes of the Atlantic coast. The sand was red from the sandstone. The wind had whipped the dunes so high that when we ran up to the top of them, we found ourselves looking down onto the tops of full-grown spruce trees. Sometimes we couldn't see the water; instead I felt the eerie sensation of being in the midst of a desert. Every year since 1988, a consortium has tried to get approval to build a multi-million-dollar tourist complex there, and so far, the locals have kept turning them down.

A patient with a badly infected gall bladder lived in the Selkirk area. Attack after attack, she refused to have it removed. Just after a heavy snowstorm, she had another attack. The roads were blocked for miles. Just getting the information across the telephone line was tedious. On the north side, where she lived, was an armed-service private line which had been installed during the war so spotters on the coast could report German submarines. After the war, it was up to the farmers along that particular route to maintain the line. They used the old wall telephones with the crank that ran on batteries, and the batteries were often weak. A message might have to be relayed through a half-dozen people to get from the north side to where we were, and the same thing on the way back. So I finally got the message about her problem.

The only way to get out there was by railway. There was a station at the end of the river, so I drove there and waited for a handcar.[4] I climbed on, and the railroad section man operated the pump to propel it forward. After about fourteen miles he let me out, and I waded through about a mile of fields. In some spots the snow came up to my hips; where it had drifted, it was closer to my armpits. By the time I reached her house I was ready to drop. All I could do was give her some medications to keep her under control until she could get to hospital, where the doctors could attend to her ruptured gall bladder.

When I reached the tracks, the section man was standing there on the handcar waiting for me. He had waited about an hour, knowing I'd need a ride back sooner or later.

You might be wondering, "Did people appreciate this kind of service?" Not necessarily; they expected it.

That spring, the roads were particularly bad. The Seven Mile Road from Dingswell Mills to the south was hopeless. The soft mud went down about three feet. I could tell by looking at the tractors; even with their six-foot wheels they had sunk down to the axles. One of my patients was a two-year-old boy who was running an extreme fever of 106 degrees and had started to convulse. In order to get to him I had to drive thirty-five miles to Charlottetown, another thirty-five miles on the other leg of the V, and then five miles in by horse and wagon. After treating him I had to return the same way. One 150 miles to make a 30-mile house call! That broke all records, but my rates hardly reflected it: fifteen dollars for the trip and five dollars for penicillin.

The main road from Charlottetown to Summerside—now the Trans-Canada Highway—was frightful. There was one particular stretch, about three hundred feet long, that took the cake. One spring, after the ground thawed out, there was so much broken pavement and mud in this spot that a stoneboat[5] was the only answer. A tractor would be stationed on each side of the highway to pull these stoneboats. We would drive onto it, and the tractor would pull us across the mud and deposit us on the other side. The only difference between these contraptions and the ones used in the fields was that these were built with heavier planks, to hold the weight of the cars. It was a slow process whenever there was traffic. Some years the pavement was completely destroyed, as the weight of the cars would smash it handily once the ground softened up. Now the roads are deeply ditched on both sides for drainage.

One morning the telephone rang and an urgent voice asked, "Can you make an emergency call?"

I said, "Yes," and the line went dead.

About an hour later I picked up the phone, and it was the same voice. "When the hell are you coming on that emergency call I telephoned about?"

"You might tell me where I'm supposed to go."

"Oh!" he said, and told me the address. Just goes to show how some people lose their heads in emergencies.

One thing that really ticked Helen off was our lack of privacy. She read a chocolate cake recipe to a friend over the phone, and shortly after she was through the telephone operator rang. "I missed a couple of the ingredients because another call came in. Would you mind repeating them?"

About eight o'clock on a Sunday morning the doorbell rang. I got out of bed, put on a robe, and went to the door. A man, dressed in his Sunday finest, stood on my front step. There was a worried look on his face. I invited him inside. When he was half in I asked, "What's the matter?"

He said with difficulty, "I have a pain in my chest." I was standing inches from him and looking into his face when his expression went blank. His pupils widened out and he slumped towards me. I instinctively held him up until I realized he had died, and then let the body fall. When I called the Glebe house to notify the priest, the housekeeper took down the information and relayed it to the priest, who was delivering a sermon at the time. Instead of coming down to the office, the priest offered prayers for the dead man during the church service—with the deceased's wife and children sitting in one of the pews! They had thought he was outside taking some air, and suddenly they were hearing his eulogy. Didn't seem the best way to notify loved ones.

Meanwhile, nobody could locate the undertaker. It was a beautiful Sunday; he might have gone fishing. I had some patients to attend to in Souris, so I left Helen there with the body sprawled across the floor. No one was authorized to touch it except the undertaker. Helen wasn't tickled about having to step over him every time the phone rang. The undertaker finally arrived in the late afternoon.

The Christmas holidays were fast approaching and we had hoped to get away to Springhill. But with four maternity cases due right around that time, we had to resign ourselves to staying put. On December 24, I was called to the hospital in Souris and delivered the first one. While I was there, I received a call from Montague Hospital that another maternity had just been admitted. As I was on my way out the front door at Souris, a nurse rushed up to me.

"Your maternity has come in, Dr. Burden," she said.

"That patient's been delivered," I said.

"Not yet," she said. "She just arrived."

So I delivered that second one, and while I was cleaning up, a call came in from a hospital in Charlottetown concerning the fourth of my maternity cases! I went on to Montague, delivered that baby, and then headed into Charlottetown. Four deliveries in five hours in three different hospitals is a record I haven't beat since. The day after Christmas, I visited all of them to see how they were doing, and then Helen, Bill, and I went on to Springhill for two days.

The 24th of May was a lovely spring day. Helen and I and Stan and Lily decided to take the kids for a picnic. We left early to beat the patients' convenient holiday arrivals. First Stan proceeded to run over my new wheelbarrow putting his truck in the garage. Then, once we had the picnic supplies and the kids in my car, we noticed half a dozen of Stan's piglets running free. Can you imagine the two of us reaching down, trying to catch them in the slippery wet grass? We caught more than the two dozen that were in the pen before we noticed two escape routes. We caught the last one about a mile from home. By then we needed a restful day, and even managed to pull away before the first patient showed up.

NOTES

1. Splenectomy: Removal of the spleen.

2. Ampoules: Vials.

3. Hurl: The iridescent part of a peacock feather.

4. Handcar: A railroad track maintenance vehicle.

5. Stoneboat: A horse-drawn sled that farmers used to clear stones from fields.

8. Surgery on a Horsehair Sofa, a Mysterious Suicide, and Murder by Mistake

After a heavy snowstorm I went out on a house call, but the car could only make it so far; I hoofed it the rest of the way. After wading through fields in waist-deep snow, the patient's son greeted me with the logical question, "Where's your car?" I gestured over yonder and went in to examine his mother's broken hip. I told him she would have to be moved to hospital for further care, and was halfway out the door when he stopped me.

"I'm taking you back by horse and sleigh," he insisted. We set out, and the horse floundered at the first heavy drift. The farmer unhitched him and led him aside. Then the two of us made a track through the drift by walking back and forth several times. After pulling the sleigh through, we re-hitched the horse on the other side and set out again. I'll be darned if we didn't have to repeat this ritual several times before we reached my car. I didn't have to be a rocket scientist to figure I'd have been much better off walking back alone, in the tracks I made on the way in.

A few weeks after that episode, a man showed up at my door with a horse and sleigh. Another snowstorm had just dumped several feet on the village, so driving was once again out of the question. Two provincial snowplows had already gotten stuck, one on the road and the other in a field. We headed south in the sleigh towards Montague. The patient, about fifty years old, was having a severe stomach hemorrhage which had been brought on by an ulcer. Every half hour he would vomit up another pan of pure blood. He couldn't be moved, so I sent his neighbour back to my office with a note to Helen. She rounded up the intravenous fluids, plasma expanders, intravenous tubing, and needles, and the fellow raced them back to me. My chief concern was to keep the patient from going into shock from loss of blood.

Since we weren't exactly in a hospital room, I had to improvise an intravenous stand. I tied a heavy-corded lobster trap head to the drapery rod and stood the IV fluid bottle upside down in the opening. Since the hemorrhaging continued through the night, the neighbour had to make several trips back to the office for supplies. Finally, just before dawn, the bleeding eased; his blood pressure had dropped from loss of blood. Since he had no phone, I went home to make arrangements to get him to hospital.

Heavy truck plows began the task of opening up the road, which was on a hill, for the ambulance. One of the drivers would gun it, hit the drift at high speed, and get stuck, and then the second one would hook on a chain and pull the first one out. Under other circumstances one would have thought they were stand-ins for Laurel and Hardy. They worked from five in the morning until two in the afternoon and ended up clearing less than a half-mile. By the time the ambulance finally arrived at the house the patient had decided not to go to hospital! One of his sons came to me with the news. I was livid. I marched out to the sleigh, the young fellow brought me back, and I stormed inside. I went up to him and said point-blank, "I'll kill you right now instead of letting you bleed to death, if you don't get on this goddamned stretcher and into the ambulance!" I told him that it was a miracle he had lived through the night.

After a few uneasy moments of silence he looked up at me and said, "Ok, Doc. Take me away." We got him to Charlottetown where whole blood was in good supply.

It was a winter of storms. Another evening at about eight o'clock a call came in from the other side of Morell, about six miles away. A man had had a stroke. This time a heavy bulldozer plow went ahead to break road and I followed behind in a maintainer plow. After two hours of driving like this in the blizzard, the first driver signalled us to stop. He got out and clambered over the snow to my driver. "I don't know where the road is," he said. "Are we in a field?"

"Haven't a clue."

"The way I figure, if we go any further we could wind up in the Midgell River." I recall not finding that comment particularly comforting. We had gone less than two miles, about a mile an hour. We about-faced and I got dropped off at home. There were so many calls coming in I had to make a list so I could attend them in order once the storm broke.

The next morning the sun was brilliant and so we started out again in the same two plows around eight o'clock. In daylight, we could stay on the road by keeping an eye on the telephone poles. By noon we had gone about four miles when a farmer came up to us on snowshoes. "My wife's got a hot meal for you inside," he said, which didn't meet with much resistance. We travelled the remaining two miles to Morell in four hours, and

I attended the patient. Later, when the snow blower plow from Summerside opened the road for car traffic, the measurement of drifts showed seventeen feet of snow in some places. The wind that had blown down the bay and across the fields had deposited avalanches of snow.

Another call during a storm, before the roads were plowed, was to look after the injured in a head-on collision that occurred on that same stretch of road. A snow plow had opened the road from the village to the accident. On the way back home, the snow began to blow with a fury, and I couldn't see ahead; the headlights were useless. My only comfort was knowing that the road was still blocked at the other end, so nobody would be coming towards me from the village. On each side there was a wall of snow that rose up several feet above the roof of the car. I rolled down my window and shone my six-volt flashlight on the snow wall a couple of feet away. I drove all the way home without looking through the windshield. My eye was glued to the wall, and that was the only time I ever had to drive looking sideways.

And then there was the call that made me wish I had taken up plumbing. On the north-side road, a man had been standing on the draw bar of a moving tractor that had the big six-foot wheels. He must have had snow under his boot, because he slipped off the bar. His face struck the treads of one of the wheels. When I got to the farm, he was laying on a horsehair sofa in the kitchen, unconscious. There was a deep laceration along the side of his head, just above his ear, across his forehead, and into the point where his eye met his nose. The tire lug had hooked him just under the eyebrow. His skull bone was damaged, with part of the bone pushing down onto the brain. He was bleeding profusely on the couch and floor, and I had no one there to assist me.

He couldn't be moved by road and no helicopters were available. So I had to do what I could, with what I had. And without electricity! So with the kerosene lamp and my trusty six-volt seal beam flashlight on the table pointing at him, I went to work. I elevated the skull fracture from where it had been impacting the brain, bringing it even with the rest of the skull. Then I sutured the lacerations and the torn upper eyelid. The next day, he was taken to Charlottetown. I was told that one of the stitches on his eyelid was a bit too snug and had to be redone, and that was all that was required. Otherwise, he made a good recovery. They don't talk about that kind of surgery in college.

A major ice storm hit that winter and the power was out for a week. The power lines that spanned the Morell and Midgell Rivers had *eight inches* of ice around them. This made them so heavy that they sagged down far enough to block the roads. A farmer on his way to Souris got fed up when his horse came face to face with the telephone lines over the road, so he solved the problem the best way he knew how. He took out a pair of pliers, cut the lines, and continued on his merry way. I don't know if he ever looked back. The first line went down with a crash, pulling the pole down with it, and so on down the line until forty of them were yanked onto the ground—a real domino effect.

In the spring when Glenn Palmer came to visit, we spent a good bit of time fishing. One of our fishing trips was interrupted by the RCMP, and not because we were breaking the law. As coroner, they asked me to investigate an apparent suicide towards the north shore. We drove up to the farmhouse and then into the back field. A young man was hanging from a spruce tree. I went up to him, quickly determined he was dead, and looked into his face as it hung from the rope. He couldn't have been more than seventeen. "Why would anybody do this?" I asked myself, stupefied. I had seen many men killed in the war, but this was not the same. I cut him down since there was no evidence of foul play, nor were there any further clues as to the cause of death.

According to his family, he had been plowing the field earlier that day. The rows started off perfectly straight, gradually became more and more staggered, and then stopped completely. That must have been the point at which he took the horse to the far end of the field, tied it to a tree, and came back down with a rope from the horse's reins. He slung the rope partway up the spruce tree, put the other end around his neck, stood on top of a fencepost, and dropped off.

He had been out the night before playing cards and his buddies said he'd seemed absolutely normal. His parents didn't notice anything out of the ordinary at breakfast either. Something happened that made those rows go crooked, and not even his family will ever know the answer.

The first time Helen and I got a babysitter for Bill, our firstborn son, it was quite a special occasion. A coronation ball was being held for Queen Elizabeth II in the village hall. Evening gowns and dark suits replaced the attire for the normal Saturday night dances. We socialized with some friends before the ball. Partway through the gala event, I was called out. There had been a shooting in Morell Rear. All I was told was that it happened in the first house past the railway tracks. Helen wanted to come with me, and we dropped by the house so I could change coats and pick up some emergency supplies. It was about eleven o'clock.

There were no lights when we crossed the railway tracks. My headlights picked up a truck through an opening in the trees, so I turned in there. A young fellow of about twenty was standing beside the truck. He seemed awfully shook up.

"Is this where the shooting occurred?" I asked.

"Yes."

"Where's the patient?"

He shot back: "He is dead."

"Well, we'd better check and find out if he is," I answered.

It was pitch black, so we had to grope our way towards the house. He entered first and headed for the kitchen, where he found a kerosene lamp. He came out into the entry hall with the flame bobbing inside the glass chamber, and he said, "He's upstairs." He pointed to the staircase with the lamp. I went on up, clutching my medical case. He followed close behind me with the lamp. I asked, "What happened?"

"I shot him."

I got a sinking feeling in my gut, knowing the killer was right behind me, but I kept my feet moving. I didn't know whether or not he still had the gun. I went in to the bedroom and examined the body; it was his father. A single bullet had entered his forehead, and there was just one drop of blood below the bullet hole.

An RCMP officer came in and asked if he could question the boy using the back seat of my car. Helen was in the front seat, but I had to say yes. As coroner, I checked through the house with another officer. Later Helen told me that the cold bothered her more than the questioning.

It turns out that the boy and his girlfriend were playing cards in the kitchen when the father came home drunk. He insulted the girl, so the boy promptly took her home and came back. The day before, a friend of his had brought over a .22 rifle with a sawed-off barrel to introduce him to target practice. This was the first time the kid had ever fired a gun. The friend left the gun behind. As this fellow explained in the court case, he took the gun upstairs and pointed it at his father, just to scare him. It went off by mistake. The gun was later tested and the hairline trigger did prove to be defective. He got fourteen years in prison—a lot of time to think about pointing loaded guns.

The irony of it is the boy was the only one in the family who got along with his father. They had just bought a truck together. The mother had been away, and showed up the day of the killing and many people in the area believed she did it and the boy was taking the rap. But this was disproven in court.

One of the families that called on my services regularly never paid. What burned me up was that they were well-to-do. It wasn't hard to tell, because they had big tractors, bailers, and plows on their farm. The lady would speak about her magazine subscriptions at the church group meetings Helen attended. Helen and I couldn't afford magazines! After two maternity cases and numerous office visits and house calls, I began sending them bills. After the sixteenth monthly bill with no response, I noticed that they were going to Charlottetown for medical care. I figured it was time for some advice. I spoke with a lawyer who knew them well and he wrote them a letter. This was as far as I ever got to suing a client for non-payment. It sure brought results, since the man not only paid my bill, but the lawyer's fee as well. Right after that they started coming to me again, and paying cash each time.

One early evening a call came in from Dingswell Mills. I drove out and parked in front of a one-bedroom tarpaper shack. An ashen-faced man in his mid-thirties was laying on a built-in bunk, gritting his teeth in pain. Bread flour had been packed all around his elbow and blood seeped through from the wound beneath.

He and his wife and child had gone to visit her father in their horse and buggy. The father-in-law came out of his house with a shotgun, and without saying a word, fired into the buggy. The load of shot caught this fellow in the elbow and blew most of the elbow away. His wife and child were unharmed. This fellow then proceeded, somehow, to drive all the way home.

As I was picking off the flour in order to cleanse the wound, I asked, "Where is this fellow who shot you?"

He replied, "Out in the woods somewhere with the gun."

The kerosene lamp was behind me and I realized what a perfect silhouette I made in the window. So I quickly moved the lamp and examined him standing off to the side. Since the bleeding had stopped, I bandaged and put a splint on the arm and took him to Souris Hospital. There I was able to take off the remaining bread flour and thoroughly examine the arm. It was a ragged shotgun wound, and the elbow bone was pretty well gone. Bones were sticking out and the ulnar nerve was laying across the wound. The lower arm was just held on by tendons, but the ulnar nerve seemed to be intact. I had an ambulance bring him to a larger hospital in Charlottetown so he could receive maximum care. I expected him to end up with a flail arm[1] but he wound up with a fairly decent elbow, which was amazing in light of how much bone he had lost.

When I got to Souris, the RCMP were notified and they were out in force looking for the father-in-law. They set up lights, surrounded his house with high-powered rifles, and ordered him through a loudspeaker to come out. The man sauntered out, rubbing his eyes. He had been asleep in his bed, which meant that he had not been out in the woods by the son-in-law's after all. Never did find out the father-in-law's motive for the shooting.

In Charlottetown, a doctor friend who was an officer in the reserve army suggested that if I joined I would have the rank of captain. So I did, and before my uniform was issued, the inspection was underway for the best medical company in Canada, so that the Ryerson-Schillington Award could be presented. The inspecting officers were told that I hadn't been issued a uniform, and so we didn't lose points on that account. We were given maps of the area and told to set up the

Field Ambulance Company. When we did this, we noticed that one side was vulnerable to shell fire. We suggested sandbags be used for protection. The inspecting officers asked where we would get the sandbags. I said, "We'll get at least empty bags from the nearest engineers' unit or RCEME.[2] In the meantime, we'll put a couple of men out on the road to get or steal some from the passing Bren gun carriers or tanks that use them for extra armour."

The inspecting officers glanced at each other. Later, in the officers' lounge, Major Gagnon, one of the inspecting officers, took me aside and asked, "How did you get that information?"

"I spent five years overseas with No. 7 Canadian General Hospital," I replied.

The next time he visited, I was wearing my uniform and had on my service ribbons. And the good news is, we won the trophy.

One evening while getting dressed to go to Charlottetown for reserve army, I got an emergency call to visit a sick child. I left wearing the uniform and had to stop the car a mile or so from the house because the mud was so deep. I travelled that last stretch of road standing on the draw bar of a tractor. At first the mother didn't know what to make of a doctor wearing a mud-spattered army medical uniform, but I must have convinced her I was for real, since she let me in.

A colonel in the Medical Corps died in Charlottetown. Since he was entitled to a full military funeral my unit was involved, and I was second-in-command of the parade. The rain, snow, and wind conspired to make it a totally miserable day. By the time we got to the church, we were all wet. The insignia bearer, who was holding the cushion displaying the medals, was covered with four inches of wet snow. With the parade standing at attention, the parade commander passed in front of me and remarked, "Only a medical officer would die and get buried on a day like this."

Of all the strange things I've seen in my medical practice, this one holds a special place in my memory. It started with a phone call from a priest.

"Hello, doctor. How can I get a death certificate? I need it so I can get a burial permit for a member of the church."

"Get it from the man's doctor," I told him.

"The man was ninety years old and hadn't seen a doctor for many years. He died at home, from old age."

So that meant he had to get it from the coroner, which was me. Now I was catching on.

We travelled about six miles up a back road and came upon a two-storey farmhouse. The priest said in a hushed voice, "Wait in the car." He went inside and about twenty-five people came strolling out, all dressed up. I realized this must be the funeral. The priest came back out and signalled for me to come in.

From the kitchen I was ushered into the middle room. There wasn't a stick of furniture in it except for two kitchen chairs facing each other, spanned by two rough two-by-eight planks. Lying on his back on the planks was the deceased, a lanky man with a white beard, dressed in a suit. His arms were folded. I had expected to see a coffin. Suddenly it dawned on me that the churchyard was next door. I discharged my duties as coroner, signed the death certificate, and on the way out looked over at the churchyard. A rough box was waiting for him at the grave site. This was the only funeral I've seen that spared the coffin.

The night of Thursday, November 1, 1956, my daily routine ended. When I came home from work, Helen told me she had heard on the radio that something serious had happened in the mines in Springhill. We took a radio to bed and heard the broadcast: "At 5:10 PM today there was an explosion and a fire in the No. 4 coal mine in Springhill. A number of dead were found on the surface. All underground miners are trapped. There is a good possibility they are dead. Draegermen Bill Ferguson and Alex Spence died trying to get into the mine. Most of the surface workers are either dead or very seriously injured." Then came the list of several miners who had died, beginning with Pleaman Pyke, my boyhood buddy.

I was in sudden, severe shock. I caught my breath, thinking, "Another schoolmate gone." I got up and packed bandages, dressings, IV equipment, and cleaned out any emergency supplies I had on hand. When I went back to bed, I set the alarm for four o'clock so I could catch the first ferry at Borden, about eighty miles away. Somehow we managed to get some sleep, and the next morning, in the black of night, I headed for Springhill.

NOTES

1. Flail arm: An arm that bends down as well as up.

2. RCEME: Royal Canadian Electrical and Mechanical Engineers.

9. The Mine Explosion: Rescuing the Trapped Men

THE SPRINGHILL MINE DISASTER OF 1956 IS A WELL-KNOWN TRAGEDY. THE EXPLOSION IN THE NO. 4 MINE THAT OCCURRED on that fateful day, the first of November, claimed the lives of thirty-nine miners. The royal commission that was established to investigate the Explosion concluded that the disaster began when a trolley of fine coal and dust went up the slope against the flow of air. This filled the air inside the mine with fine explosive dust. Before the trolley was unloaded at the surface, some of the empty coal cars broke free, ran back down the slope, and jumped the rails. One of the wayward cars slammed into a power line, causing it to arc. The spark ignited the explosive airborne dust at the 5500 level, which blew up the slope and towards the surface, where the additional oxygen fuelled a heat blast that killed the workers and destroyed the bankhead.[1] The timbers were blown a couple of hundred feet into the air and the heat was so intense that they spontaneously caught fire in mid-air on the way down. The explosion was heaviest on the surface where there were greater concentrations of airborne dust and oxygen.

This was one of the gravest mining disasters in North American history. What follows is my own first-hand account of the rescue effort, which I have reconstructed from the notes I made underground and shortly afterwards. The media certainly covered the story, but many of the fine points were lost to reporters who had never set foot in the mine. For example, the draegermen[2] were the only reported heroes. In fact, they were few in number compared to the barefaced miners who didn't hesitate to go below into the after-damp[3] without protection in order to locate and rescue their trapped fellow workers.

The twenty-five-year-old No. 4 mine was situated on the western end of Main Street. The baseball diamond and the baseball, softball, and soccer fields were north of the street that ran to the mine. The No. 2 and No. 4 mines were adjacent. The slopes went underground to the west at approximately a thirty degree angle, following the natural coal seam, and the two mines shared the same horseshoe-shaped bankhead.

When I arrived at the mines I didn't even think of going underground to join in the rescue. By that time there were plenty of draegermen and experienced miners from the coalfields of Nova Scotia. But I had handled large numbers of casualties during the war. And now that I was a doctor, and these were my friends in my own hometown, I was here to help. Plus, I was familiar with the No. 4 mine, having worked there during my second summer in college.

My first stop was the hospital, but there wasn't much I could do there either. The miner-patients who had been on the bankhead at the time of the explosion were either dead or dying. A nurse called me over to determine if a certain patient was still alive. He wasn't, and I had to ask who it was. "Les Nelson," she replied. Les had sat with me in school; I had known him all my life. Yet here he was, laid out on the lily-white hospital sheets, totally unrecognizable. His skin was like hardened leather, burned to a crisp. I tensed up, beginning to wonder how many more of

The 1956 Explosion in No. 4 Mine

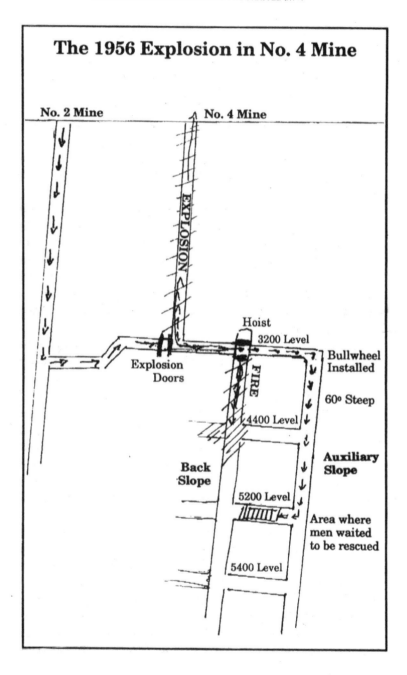

my friends and relations would meet this horrible fate. And was there any hope whatsoever for getting the men out who were unaccounted for? This was the third classmate of mine out of the first half-dozen to die from the explosion. I helped load two other severe burn cases onto stretchers so they could be flown to the Victoria General Hospital in Halifax. Even with the most expert care, they both died the following week.

Radios blared non-stop, broadcasting the Russian invasion of Hungary. One of the nurses, who had been born in Hungary and had come to Canada as a child, complained, "We need more news of our miners!"

It was still impossible for the rescue workers to progress underground because the gases were so strong. But something was happening on the surface to give us hope. The air compressor[4] gauges would drop, and then go back up again. This indicated that the lines, in fact, weren't broken; the old miners figured that someone down there must be turning on air valves, and then turning them off. This was the first sign of life from below, and our spirits soared. In the area where the men were believed to be trapped, there were compressed air outlet valves every three hundred feet.

By noon on Saturday, draeger teams[5] had made it to the 3400 level and reported a fire there that stopped their progress. The news media kept announcing that the miners must be dead, and they were soon proven to be false experts. None of us Springhillers would give up hope until every last man was accounted for. And the compressor gauges were already telling us a different story.

While I was at the hospital, amazing news came across the radio: Charlie Burton and Dick Ward had made it to the surface alive. MacKenzie Flemming, a draeger instructor from North Sydney, had been at the 3500 level when he heard their voices and saw their lights. Charlie and Dick carried with them the greatest news of all: fifty other miners were still alive at the 5400 level! They had holed up in a section of the level that underground manager Con Embree had protected from the gases by draping layers of brattice cloths[6] to close off a length of the level. Con had cut holes in a small compressed-air hose so each of the men could breathe when the killing gasses of the explosion backed into the level. Since the telephone lines were in the main slope where the explosion had been, communication from the surface had been cut off.

Once Charlie and Dick told their story, there was a new feeling of exhilaration. Draegermen and barefaced men headed into the deadly gasses with renewed determination.

After Charlie and Dick were brought into the All Saints Hospital, I received word that DOSCO wanted a doctor at the bankhead. I volunteered since I was already prepared with emergency supplies in my coat pocket. But first I went in to see Charlie. He was filthy dirty; his miner's clothes and face were black. By then he was breathing all right, since he had had fifteen minutes or so of air by the time he got to hospital. I then went over to the mine.

It was obvious I wasn't needed on the surface. One of the officials came over to me and said, "You could be useful down in the mines. The ones coming up are badly affected by gas." He was referring to both the trapped men and the barefaced rescuers. I was a bit anxious, knowing there was fire and gas below, but realized I was at no more risk than the others who were already down there. I knew there was a fresh-air base 2,200 feet below the surface, and that beyond that, it was dangerous. Suddenly I felt ridiculous in my blue blazer, grey flannel pants, and white shirt and tie so I disappeared and came back wearing coveralls, boots, a miner's hat with a lamp, and a belt to hold the battery.

My first step onto the slope brought back memories as I breathed in the old familiar mine smell and felt the cool air on my skin. With my emergency medical case in hand, I proceeded down the No. 2 slope to the explosion doors that separated the No. 2 from the No. 4 mine's slopes. I was the first doctor down in the mines, and anxious as I was to help, I wasn't able to go any further onto the No. 4 mine slope. The gas was overpowering, and the back slope of the No. 4 mine was closed off. The rescue operation was taking place on the auxiliary slope—the slope I had travelled back to the surface one day during the miners' summer vacation in 1948 when the manrake was out of order. At that time only five men were working, and two of them would die in this disaster.

I made it to the fresh air base almost a half-mile down. Both the rescuers and the men being rescued were using oxygen tanks. A draegerman on his way to the surface gave me a partly used oxygen cylinder, and I moved along the level with John Phalean to assist the miners. Since it was just a tank with a valve, I had to cup my hands simultaneously over the slightly opened valve and the man's nose and mouth until he was revived enough to be moved from the fresh-air base to the surface. Beyond the fresh-air base, the gas filled the level to within a foot or so from the floor. I came upon one fellow who was collapsing from the poisonous gas and gave him oxygen. I didn't recognize him, and said to myself, "Who's this bird? I don't know him." When he revived, I said, "You'd better get to the surface." Then I noticed blueprints in his pocket and asked who he was. Meanwhile, he was asking someone else who the hell I was. Finally I was introduced to the chief engineer from DOSCO, Mr. Haslem.

When he was told I was a doctor, he said, "If you say I must go, I will, but I'm needed down here." Since he had inhaled a lot of gas I instructed him to go to the fresh-air base. That way he could still be on hand in the mine.

I continued along the tunnel[7] trying to revive men who had fallen down from the gas. By this time we were crawling on our bellies since the only breathable air was within a foot and a half of the floor. Soon we came to the end of the tunnel and began treating men at the head of the auxiliary slope. A draeger team was rigging a bull wheel[8] so that a trolley could be used to get the men up the "steep."[9]

From where I was I could see a trapped man heading up the slope and then collapsing. A rescuer who went after him also collapsed. Soon there were four down, but then the gas seemed to lift and they were able to make it to the fresh-air base where we revived them before sending them on to the surface.

Walk-around masks had been sent in by the Royal Canadian Air Force. They were designed for use in high-flying aircraft to enable the men to move about in air that had low oxygen content. The barefaced men didn't understand their intended use, and so they were trying to stand up in the gas, thinking they were protected. They would get extra oxygen, and along with it a heavy dose of toxic gasses. I began to tape the sides of the masks so that only oxygen was able to get through. Until we were able to send word to the surface to prepare these masks properly, rescuers were falling down right and left.

I was trying to revive one man, lying on my stomach in the tunnel and holding a mask over his face. Someone brought another semi-conscious man up beside him. Both were unconscious but still breathing. I transferred the walk-around oxygen mask from one hand to the other, and then had to raise up my head onto the first fellow's chest in order to get an oxygen mask over the second man's face. Suddenly my head seemed to grow bigger—and bigger—and bigger until it finally seemed to explode. I went unconscious, my head rolling over and down into a low spot in the floor. The air was reasonably good there and I soon came to. My first coherent thought was: "My God, I'm down here and if I don't make it back up I've got a wife and children who will have nothing. At least compensation will look after the families of the miners who are down here, but I'm not covered by compensation or anything else. In fact, I'm not even being paid!" But I still had two men to revive, and so got back to work, careful to keep my head close to the floor.

The trapped men were telling us how many more were coming behind them. When the gas got worse, we all figured no one else would be coming, so I went back up to the surface for something to eat and a few hours' sleep. I had been down in the mine for about eight hours.

By this time, thirty-six of the trapped men had been rescued. By stopping along the way for air at the compressed air valves and getting oxygen from the rescuers, they were able to make it to the fresh-air base, and from there to the surface.

One of the draegermen who had come up from the rescue asked my mother-in-law if she knew where I was.

"Oh, he's at the hospital," she said.

"No, no," he said. "He's down in the mine."

She wasn't too thrilled by that update.

After a short rest, I went back down the mine, but the mine officials told me to go back to the surface. They knew I had been knocked out by the gas and wanted to save me for later. "Wait until we reach the fifty trapped men at the 5400 level," the mine manager said. A fire was burning out of control at the 3400 level, using up oxygen and giving off carbon monoxide and carbon dioxide, which prevented access. Until that was brought under control, I sat in the manager's office, half dozing and half ready to whip into action on a moment's notice.

I missed Pleaman's funeral on Sunday because I felt I could be more useful in the rescue work. Everything was happening so fast—some men were dying while others were being saved. There wasn't much time to reflect on the loss of my boyhood friends—there was time for that later.

At 5:10 on Sunday morning, a five-man draeger team finally made it through to the 5400 level. When the first draegerman hollered through the brattice cloth, the trapped men didn't want to open it up for fear of letting in the gas. I was alerted, and along with Dr. Roy Munroe, another Springhiller who had been best man at my wedding, went down through the tunnel to the auxiliary slope. Roy was needed somewhere along the way, so I went on alone into the area where the trapped men were. Barefaced men were there to guide me. There were four doctors below the fresh-air base, three of whom were from Springhill and had become doctors after the war. Another eighteen doctors were either at the fresh-air base or on their way down to it by that time.

When I lifted the brattice cloth, the men were yelling and speaking all at once. They told me Dougie Beaton was in bad shape and Dr. Buddy Condy was trying to revive him. Dougie, who had been unconscious for many hours, was lying in a cement box, and Buddy was attending him, but with no success. Dougie was very dehydrated and badly in need of iv fluids. I told Buddy, "Send to the surface and tell them what you need." Buddy sent word up for iv fluids and I went to look after some of the other men. Then I came upon Con Embree, a veteran of two previous explosions. He was stareyeyed, clutching his hands across his chest, and breathing in short gasps. I could tell he had had a coronary, but he kept moving about, checking on the men. This was the man who had saved the others by cutting holes in the compressed-air hose. I tried to quiet him down. Two of my neighbours, Bob and Lennie Smith, were also there. Bob was having chest pains. I had brought along a small bottle of rum and pulled it out of my case when I saw him, figuring he needed a bit of stimulation. After a couple of swallows, Bob remarked, "I've drunk a lot of stuff in my day, but this is the best I've ever tasted!" Except for special cases like Bob who needed immediate stimulation, we fed them gradually: first water, then hot soup, and later coffee. I determined that six men would have to be carried up the slope on stretchers.

Just then a draegerman came in and asked me to come out to the main slope, where the explosion had been. I followed him out to where some of the men were slumped against the wall ,while others lay face down on the pavement. Their lips were bright red, which told me they had been poisoned by carbon monoxide. I checked one of the officials I had worked with during the miners' vacation, and then one of my schoolmates. They were both stiff with rigor mortis. I didn't even have time to react. The IV fluid we needed for Dougie appeared, but it was just a bottle with no needle and tubing to administer it! So we sent up a more explicit message, and finally Buddy was able to give Dougie the IV fluid and oxygen, and Dougie slowly began to come around. All of the men were extremely happy to see us, but at the same time they were anxious to get to the surface. I knew the top priority was to get the six men requiring stretchers up first, with the stretchers being passed up non-stop. By this time there were over one hundred rescue workers lining the slopes. One set of six would hand a stretcher to the next six, and so on until it arrived at the surface.

While we were formulating these plans, Mr. Haslem, the engineer I had met earlier, approached me. "I want to show you something. Keep it quiet," he said. "A messenger just arrived directly from the surface and this is what he handed me." He passed me a note, saying, "See what you think."

EVACUATE THE MINE WITH ALL POSSIBLE HASTE.

I searched his eyes for a further clue, and finally burst out, "These men are weak. We can't push 'em out in a hurry. We'll move 'em just as fast as we can." I knew something was radically wrong, but I didn't know what. Nor did he. Someone up there did. The thought of another calamity was frightening, but we were too busy to be nervous. Ten men were still unaccounted for. A draeger team went down to the 5700 level and found them—all lying face down on the rock floor. One of the bodies moaned as he was moved by a draegerman who was trying to identify him. Two of the men were still alive, and the draeger team brought them to the 5400 level. We were able to revive them with oxygen, but they were still semi-conscious. Buddy or I shouted out, "We need two more stretchers, right away!" We kept giving them oxygen until they were breathing on their own in a semi-conscious state. The rescue continued as men from the first group were passed up the level on stretchers. On the "steep," which was the area with a sixty-degree slope, the makeshift bull wheel was in place so the stretchers were carefully raised up one at a time to the next level.

While all this was going on, Buddy and I sat with the two semi-conscious men, waiting for the final stretchers to be sent down. We sat there a long time. I began thinking about that note. "What did they mean?" I kept wondering. "What more could happen?"

Buddy asked, "Do you think they've forgotten we're here?"

I remembered he had never worked in the mines, and, considering his jumpiness, figured I'd better not tell him about the note. I assured him they knew we were here, and kept my concerns to myself. When I walked out of our makeshift resting place I saw a message chalked in large letters on a big galvanized metal structure just a few yards away:

NOV 4TH 1954

AT 3:30 PM

SO FAR MEN ARE IN GOOD SHAPE WE ARE ALL INSIDE
THE NO. 2 DOOR SO FOR GOD SAKE COME

EMILE MELANSON

As soon as the last two men were taken up on stretchers, Buddy and I followed. We were the last ones out of the mine area where the trapped men had been. Now that everyone was accounted for we could all breathe easier, especially after we made it to the surface! After twelve hours underground, I hit the surface with a parched throat and sucked in the sweet air of the atmosphere. Immediately I felt the glare of floodlights. The sea of townspeople was overwhelming. A hundred-bed tent had been set up by the mine entrance. Ambulances, station wagons, first aid supplies, doctors, soldiers, and newsmen all waited. The B Company of the North Nova Scotia Highlanders had taken charge of traffic control within an hour of the explosion, and worked twenty-four hours a day until we came out of the mine. Tents had been set up all over the grounds. I turned in my lamp and headed straight for my mother-in-law's for another meal and a bed.

Con Embree's personal account of the underground night-mare, as recorded in his diary, was published in the *Springhill Record* on November 8, 1954. Con's first entry was made at 9:40 PM, five hours after the explosion: "Some air and fumes are coming out of the 5400 tunnel...Smoke fumes and after-damp are coming in from the slope...We have forty-seven men here between the door and the tunnel. We have erected a stopping in the outside end of the tunnel and a stopping across the 5400 foot level just outside the tunnel and left an opening about three by five feet to let the compressed air in. We are using the air from a six-inch line to survive."

At 2:00 AM, he wrote: "Got out to the 5400 bottom. After-damp bad, but seemed to be improving some. Found Doug Beaton about twenty-five feet below the 5400 back slope bottom and got him inside of door. Very little sign of life. Applied artificial respiration. He showed some sign of recovery by 3:15 AM with men taking turns keeping up the artificial respiration, [which] we carried on...for about four hours."

At 7:30 PM on Friday, Con went back out to the 5400 bottom and found Charlie Burton collapsed on the slope. He took Charlie into the safety of the room and recorded that the men were "fairly well, but growing weaker."

At 5:15 AM on Saturday, Con ventured out to the 5400 bottom again, found five men clustered there, and brought them back to the "room." According to Con, there were as many as sixty-three men in the room at one time. "I thought the air was weakening and the men questioned if workmen were not sealing the mine. I said we are not beat yet. If some of you men will come out with me we will get the two-and-one-half inch [diameter] rubber hose used at the bottom to convey compressed air to the machinery. We brought the hose in and hooked it on the fitting on the six-inch line. Then we cut a hole in the hose for each man on opposite sides, a foot or so apart, to ensure that each man got an equal share of the compressed air."

Since the air seemed to be weakening, Con held a conference with several of the men, and they decided to try to reach the surface with the message that many of the men were safe, but that their lives depended on the compressed air supply. Charlie Burton, Harold Tabor, and George Stonehouse left the group and headed for the surface. By stopping for air every several hundred feet at the compressed-air fittings along the airway return, and with bulldog determination, the men finally reached the rescue crew.

To put the fires out, the mine was then sealed so that the oxygen could be cut off. Some months later it was reopened and the dead bodies were removed for burial. All told, thirty-nine men died in the explosion and eighty-eight were rescued. It's ironic to think back on the media's early predictions that "all are most likely dead."

The dry cleaners managed to do wonders to my grey flannel slacks and blue blazer, but I still wouldn't recommend wearing them for pit clothes. I had my family and my medical practice to attend to, so I returned to Prince Edward Island as soon as I had a) breathed enough air, b) eaten enough food, and c) gotten enough sleep.

My first patient in St. Peter's Bay was a potato farmer by the name of Mr. Squires. I was literally crawling out of my skin as I sat there listening to him say how much more dangerous farming is than coal mining! I don't remember my reply, but it wasn't nearly as good as what I came up with afterwards. Shortly after that I was invited to speak about the disaster to the Gyro Club in Charlottetown. They seemed to be a lot more enlightened than Mr. Squires.

That winter I got fed up with the driving conditions, the lack of entertainment in our small village, and the poor prospects for Bill's schooling in St. Peter's Bay. We decided to move back to Springhill. It was the natural place to go since both Helen and I had grown up there. Not being clairvoyant, neither of us knew what disasters awaited us there.

For me, the school system was probably the final straw. Bill was five and almost ready for first grade. As chairman of the school board, I knew there was nothing I could do to improve conditions. The school was just too small. There were only fifty children altogether, and six grades met in one room! Besides that, driving 22,000 miles a year on house and hospital calls had become too much of a good thing. And being on staff at four hospitals in three different directions made it impossible for me to pay daily visits to my patients.

When we decided to move, Helen and I had to go to Charlottetown to mail letters and make phone calls; otherwise the news would have become common knowledge in our village. At that time, the No. 2 Springhill mine was the deepest working mine in North America, so employment back home was brisk. I signed a contract to work at the Springhill Medical Centre for eight thousand dollars a year, much less than I had been making at my practice in Prince Edward Island. But I wouldn't have to carry medications, driving would be minimal, and I wouldn't be getting any more uninvited guests—er, patients—at my home during mealtimes.

Eight months after our second son, Kent, was born, I was carrying him down the stairs one morning. Suddenly his body stiffened, he uttered a sharp cry, and then came diarrhoea. I spoke with the doctor in Charlottetown who reassured me this was probably the stomach flu that was prevalent at that time. I didn't think so. Helen and I didn't waste any time driving him into Charlottetown, thirty-five miles away. Almost as soon as we arrived, Kent was operated on for an intussusception.[10] He lost five inches of his small bowel and half his large bowel, which had gone gangrenous due to loss of blood supply.

Helen and I stayed by his crib for days, along with special nurses. At times he stopped breathing, and we would have to give him intravenous medications instantly. After too long a time for all of us, he suddenly tried to stand up and pick the Medical Corps crest from my blazer. Looking after any child who is dangerously sick is heart-wrenching enough, but when it's your own, that adds another dimension. Once the ordeal had passed Helen and I realized that we had many pictures of our first born but almost none of Kent during those first eight months he had been with us.

NOTES

1. Bankhead: The surface structure that receives the coal from the mines. It contains washing and sorting facilities and dispenses the coal to either rail cars or trucks.

2. Draegermen: Specially trained mine rescue workers who wear self-contained breathing apparatus.

3. After-damp: Mine gasses.

4. Air compressor: Compressors ran underground equipment, such as chipper picks and small engines.

5. Brattice cloth: Tar impregnated canvas used to control ventilation in the mine.

6. The tunnel: In the No. 4 mine it was a six-foot high, six-foot wide stone walkway that had been blasted through the rock.

7. Draeger team: Five draegermen.

8. Bull wheel: A five-foot iron wheel with a steel cable for dropping down a trolley, which could then be hauled back up by a tugger engine.

9. The "steep": A sixty degree auxiliary slope that was ordinarily climbed on ladders.

10. Intussusception: The bowel turns in and digests itself.

10. *The Fire that Gobbled Up Main Street*

THE DISASTER HAD HAD A POSITIVE EFFECT ON ONE THING IN SPRINGHILL: THE PRICE OF HOUSES. WE BOUGHT AN OLDER home very much to our liking in a lovely part of town and immediately set about the necessary cleaning and painting. We were glad to be back among friends, and I was working with doctors I knew well. Dr. D. W. Fisher had been a classmate of mine in college. He, Dr. Murray and I did surgeries practically every morning for tonsillitis, appendicitis, hernias, broken bones requiring internal plating, and any number of other injuries. Open bone work was not at all unusual, which required cutting down to the bone, inserting a plate, and then setting the bone with screws through the plate.

Meanwhile, we discovered that our house on the Island that we had rented to a doctor was no longer rented. This didn't take a private detective to figure out; our rent cheques stopped coming in. The doctor had built his own house several miles away and quietly moved out. When we put it up for sale, the Lion's Club of St. Peter's Bay offered us three thousand dollars. Our real estate agent advised us not to take a penny under six thousand.

The house would get broken into, boarded up, and broken into again. I finally got fed up and went over to find out what was going on. When I walked inside, I felt like I was entering the wrong ending to a movie. Every light fixture and light switch had been removed, and the boards from the hardwood floor in the living room were stacked against the wall. Any minute I expected someone to show up with a truck and start loading. Someone was conveniently building a house, and using my house for materials! The RCMP wouldn't be bothered, so I sold the house and one acre of land to someone from out of town for one thousand dollars cash, and good riddance. So much for listening to that realtor's advice.

All Saints Hospital was squeezed by rising costs and lack of income in the days before a government hospitalization plan. We had to improvise a great deal of our equipment. For traction, we would mount pulleys over the bed and rig a makeshift apparatus from plaster, rope, and sandbags. Some of the chrome-plated instruments should have been replaced long ago, since much of the chrome had worn off. We didn't have suctions to use in case of frequent vomiting, such as people with ulcers or during stomach operations, so we would hang two gallon jugs on poles and run tubing. As the water level dropped in one bottle, the pressure would cause suction in the other. Primitive, but it worked.

The elevator was hand-operated by means of a pulley system. Nurses "man-handled" oxygen tanks weighing as much as themselves over to the bedsides. Since different sections had been built on to the hospital, the floor was rarely level. Frequently the nurses would have to cross a battlefield of ramps and varying floor heights in order to get the tank to the patient's bedside.

Despite all this, the doctors and nurses were very dedicated to their patients. We often heard patients who had been treated at newer, larger hospitals say how glad they were to return to All Saints in Springhill.

The night after Christmas 1957, I crawled into bed weary after a full day's work, and promptly fell asleep. The distinctive sound of the town's steam fire whistles brought me to in the blackness of night. I harkened back to when I had to count the whistle blows for my father when he was a volunteer fireman. Our town was divided into three wards which were indicated by either one, two, or three long blows. Then followed the short blows—up to nine, depending on the location of the fire within the ward. I counted twenty-three, two long ones and three short ones, which put the fire at the corner of Elm and Drummond streets in the area of Main Street, about one-and-a-half blocks away.

I jumped out of bed and threw the drapes back. Sure enough, the red glow lit up the night sky like a fireball. I threw on the first clothes I could find and ran down to the fire. The Stedman's Five and Dime store was engulfed in flames. As I was standing in the middle of Main Street, just down from the fire, it seemed to explode as it jumped across Main Street to Morris Saffron's three-storey furniture and clothing store on the opposite side. All three Springhill fire trucks were there, but they were dwarfed by the inferno. When it leapt across the street, it began to rage out of control, and this drove the firemen out of Stedman's. The fire quickly surrounded one of the fire trucks, which was driven out of there pronto.

Near-hurricane winds lifted large chunks of wood, tar, and asphalt shingles off the burning buildings and carried them in a vortex of smoke and flame over the roofs of adjacent stores to the residential areas of Fir Street and beyond. That was when I decided to go home and change into old clothes so I could help. Ringing up the All Saints Hospital, I got a dead line, and found out why when I got back to Main Street. The fire had burned through the electric lines on Main Street, forcing Nova Scotia

Power to kill the town's power supply. I groped in the dark for what I thought were my work clothes, laced up my boots, and headed back to the fire.

Without power, no water could be pumped into the boilers of the heating plant at the hospital. There would also be precious little water there, with so many fire trucks tying into the hydrants. The doctors would only be able to handle minor injuries; surgeries would have to be sent elsewhere. These were some of the thoughts that were racing through me. When the Oxford and Amherst fire departments arrived, the blaze was at its height. Later, Parrsboro, civil defense from Dieppe, and Pictou came on the scene with further reinforcements.

The frustration of fighting this fire came from the sad fact that the water pressure decreased as the fire grew in intensity. More and more people appeared on their roofs with hoses, and with each additional hook-and-ladder, the demand on the water supply increased. By this time, fourteen streams were on the fire. The pressure dropped from the norm of between fifty and seventy-five pounds to five pounds. When the power was restored after a couple of hours, the water supply had been so badly depleted that it remained ineffective to fight the blaze.

I ran into James Fraser, my brother-in-law, and we went over to Fir Street to his parents' home, which was in the line of the fire. The grass in the fields beyond Fir Street was already catching from the flying bits of burning debris that had blown nearly a half-mile. We organized about twenty young people to stay under cover most of the time, but also to put out the grass fires as they started, using wet sacks, mats, and sticks. Some of the flying masses of flame weighed twenty pounds or more, but the kids stuck with it in spite of their fear.

Sections of roofing were blown in the other direction, to King and Queen streets. The roof of a back kitchen on Queen

Street caught fire and we were able to put it out with a wet, moldy rug I had found lying in the field. As I was walking away, a flaming chunk of asphalt about a foot square stuck onto the back side of my hunting jacket, knocking me to the ground. I was getting up to peel the jacket off so I could throw it down and smother it when a stream of ice-cold water drenched me. The force pushed me about four feet ahead. A nearby fire truck had saved me, but now I had cold water running under my shirt and pant legs, and filling up my boots. Someone came over and picked the stuck shingle off my jacket where the tar had melted into the fabric.

Since the young people seemed to be controlling the flying embers, I went back to Fir Street where the Charles O'Brien house was on fire. This wooden-frame, two-storey home had had a hole burnt through its roof by a previous fire, and had been vacant ever since. It was directly behind Morris Saffron's store, so a lot of flaming debris had fallen inside. Next door was Charles Wilson's house, just a few feet away. Wilson's son-in-law, Bill Graven Jr., was standing between the buildings with a garden hose, trying to reach his father-in-law's roof. The pitiful stream of water only made it up about ten feet, which was halfway. I relieved him by kneeling down with my back to the fire and covering it with the wet rug I had been carrying around. Soon the fire broke through the wall behind me and I began to smell the smoking rubber of my boots, so I got out of there in a hurry. Both of those houses ended up total losses.

We moved around to the opposite side of the Wilson house, broke through a window, and I sprayed the hose down into the basement to keep the oil tanks wet while Bill began carrying furniture out onto the lawn. Soon there were about fifteen of us, and we managed to clear the house out before it gave up the ghost. I had left my typing and shorthand books on the basement window ledge of this house sixteen years before, when I was a student in night school.

About this time, one of the Springhill fire trucks pulled up next door, dropped off a fireman, and hooked into the Elgin Street hydrant. I helped hold the hose for him, but the pressure still wasn't great enough to reach the roof. Meanwhile, the nozzle was leaking so badly that almost as much water leaked out the back as sprayed through the front. It ran into all my pockets, down the inside of my pants, and bubbled out the tops of my boots. I was shivering so much I could hardly hold the hose. That was when I threw in the towel; at about five o'clock I went home for a hot toddy, a bath, and some sleep. As I fell off to sleep, I wondered how a town could go on with one disaster after another, but was thankful that this time there had been no loss of life. With the precious gift of daylight in the morning I discovered that my "work clothes" from the night before had included my best pair of blue serge pants.

The fire was finally brought under control at seven o'clock and heavy rains helped to finish it off. One fireman was admitted to hospital for smoke inhalation; otherwise, there were no injuries. But the tally of damages was grim. Four houses, two apartments, and fourteen businesses burned to the ground. The total loss was well over a million dollars, leaving thirty-four people homeless and about seventy-five without jobs.

Businesses lost included a photographic studio, an insurance company, a variety store, two clothing stores, a shoe store, the *Springhill Record* newspaper office, a furniture and clothing store, a grocery store, a hardware store, a millinery store, a mail-order catalogue office, and a barber shop. A big chunk of the heart of downtown Springhill.

11. *The Bump: Burial or Nightmare*

LESS THAN A YEAR LATER, ON OCTOBER 23, 1958, THE MOST SEVERE BUMP IN NORTH AMERICAN MINING HISTORY DEVAS-tated the people of Springhill. The No. 2 mine was 14,200 feet deep—about two and a half miles into the bowels of the earth. The main slope went down 7,800 feet where a tunnel joined it to the back slope, which went the rest of the way down. The men worked a nine-foot-high coal seam along the walls, in between the levels.[1] Since much of the slope was double tracked, an electric hoist on the surface could raise up the coal while sending the men empty boxes below in one operation.

The provincial government had established the royal commission on the Acadian Coal Company in 1937 to determine the cause of bumps. Also known as the Carroll Commission, it reported the following in 1939:

> *The strata consists of strong shale and sandstone and this strong strata permits the total extraction of the No. 2 coal even at the depth without undue maintenance of road-ways, however the strong strata are causes of other serious operational problems.*
>
> *Stresses thrown upon them by the removal of coal are not immediately released but are built up until they reach*

such magnitude that in the room and the pillar system,[2] the pillars disintegrate instantly and what is known as a "bump" occurs.

For this reason the system of work in the No. 2 colliery was changed about twenty years ago from room and pillar to the long wall retreating.[3]

Since that time [1939] "bumps" have not been as frequent but in recent years the incidence of upheavals again occurred and during the United Mine Workers' convention in Truro, No. 2 Mine was "tied-up" because of a dispute resulting from a production cutback so that the walls could be lined up.

At the time of the Bump, coal was being mined on the three walls between the 12,600 level and the 13,800 level, and then shovelled onto the pan line. The pan was shaken by an engine, which forced the coal to slide downhill to the level below where it either went onto conveyors or into boxes. From there it was taken out to the slope and sent up to the surface. Day shift ran from 7:00 AM to 3:00 PM, afternoon shift from 3:00 PM to 11:00 PM, and night shift from 11:00 PM to 7:00 AM. The mine worked non-stop. The night of the Bump, there were 174 men working underground. At that time, the walls were practically in line, one above the other, and about 1,700 feet from the slope. The miners were using the retreating wall method, so they worked towards the slope and allowed the roofs of the furthermost mined areas to fall in as they set up packs in the freshly mined section. Picture the miner. Furthest from him is the waste, where the roof has been purposely allowed to fall in. Then there are a set of packs holding up the roof where the coal has been removed. Then comes the travelling road[4] between the rows of packs alongside the wall, then

another pack, and finally the pan line just before the coal face.
WASTE – PACKS—TRAVELLING ROAD—PACK—PAN LINE—COAL
FACE.

Before the men go into the mine, they change into their
pit clothes and go to the lamp cabin to exchange metal discs
for their lamps and batteries. The metal disc and the lamp bear
the same number, so that in an emergency a mine official can
quickly tally who is in the mine by counting the discs on the
board in the lamp cabin. Also, God forbid, if someone is crushed
beyond recognition in a disaster, he can be identified by the
number on his battery.

The Springhill miners were steady workers and there were
few disruptions due to strikes or illegal walkouts. The miners on
the wall worked cooperatively since they were paid according to
the amount of coal that reached the surface during their shift.
Overall, the men were a jolly group, and even though they were
conscious of the dangers surrounding them, they seldom let on.
On the way down the slope, they'd joke and rib each other, or
comment on the latest hockey or ball game. If the pan lines
stopped for some reason while they were working on the walls,
they'd pick up again with their lighthearted bantering. This is
how the men lived with their jobs, knowing full well that they
could meet with sudden injury or death at any moment.

On October 23, 1958, a small bump occurred during the
evening shift, but no one was injured and work continued as
usual. In fact, the men were glad because small bumps relieved
some of the pressure that had built up in the mine, making the
chances of a serious bump more remote. After the small bump at
7:00 PM, the men working on the coal face began to notice how
much easier it was to remove the coal, as if a hidden pressure
were pushing it out. At 8:06 PM, the most convulsive bump in local mining history filled in the open spaces in the underground

maze, particularly at the walls. It severely impacted the middle of the three walls that were being mined, and the ends of the four levels nearest the walls.

I was in my office at the medical centre on Main Street, about a quarter of a mile away. Dr. Fisher, Dr. Murray, and I were on duty, along with a nurse and a receptionist. A patient had just left my office when the building shook. I felt three distinct shock waves, like a stick of bombs being dropped from a fighter bomber, exploding just fractions of a second apart. We all knew from the magnitude of the impact that it was a major disaster in the mines. I walked out into the hall just as one of the girls ran up the stairs and burst in. She raced up to our nurse, who was her sister, crying, "My God, Wes is down there!" (Wes was her husband.) We closed up the office in no time, and the other doctors headed up to the hospital as I drove down to the mines.

The whole town had been shaken. Many said it felt like a transport truck had plowed into the side of their homes. People felt it fifteen miles away in Amherst. According to scientific instruments in Halifax and Dartmouth, the Bump resembled a small earthquake. The shock waves took seventeen seconds to travel the 150 miles to the cities.

Unlike other emergencies in the mines, no whistles blew this time; it wasn't necessary. The whole town headed for the mine area, some to help, but many just plain anxious about the men who were underground. I went straight to the mine manager's office and asked George Calder if there was anything I could do to help.

"There's probably going to be," he answered. "We don't know just what happened down there yet. I don't want you going down until we find out. Just stay handy here on the surface."

No one was answering the telephone at the back slope, so the surface was totally cut off from the mine. I sat down in a corner of the office while the mine manager organized a group of twenty barefaced men who were willing to brave the possible dangers. And then he took them down.

Before long we got the word. The barefaced men saw miners' lamps on the back slope near the 13,400 level. By this time the coal-rakes had been replaced by man-rakes. I went into the wash house and changed into a miner's outfit. Shortly after nine o'clock I went down on a rake with two draeger teams. Since I wasn't an employee of the coal company, a mine official had to come with me, and they sent Dan O'Rourke. Three of us were barefaced—Dan, myself, and the trip driver—and the ten draegermen wore their breathing apparatus.

The gas was different from the gas after the Explosion. This time there was no carbon monoxide. In the tunnel to the back slope, our lamps reflected a good deal of light off the coal and wood on either side. That was where we saw the first miners. There were about a dozen of them. Some limped, some held their arms, some had obvious leg and back injuries, some were bleeding from their faces. They helped each other walk. Pete Amon, my stepmother's brother, was among them. It goes without saying that their faces were black. But fear was evident in the eyes of some. I asked if anyone needed emergency treatment. Getting no reply, I turned to Pete and said, "Are you all right?"

He nodded and kept on going. After a few steps he turned around and warned: "It's very bad down there."

That was all I needed to hear. When a miner says it's bad, look out.

We made it to the back-slope rake and headed down. After a short while, the men's safety lamps[5] went out. Attempts to relight them failed. This meant the gas was getting heavy. As one of the barefaced men, my palms were sweaty.

The 1958 Bump in No. 2 Mine

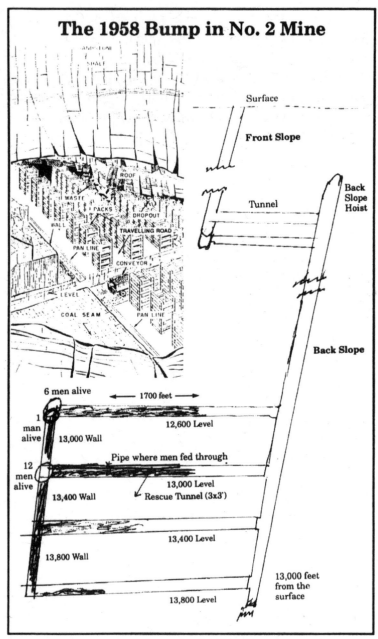

Dark areas show damaged areas.

The air was better in the level and up the 13,800 wall. I kept wondering just what we would find. Far too few men had passed us on the way to the surface. In the No. 4 mine, gas[6] and fire had been the main hazards. Here, we had been told, miners had been crushed inside the walls. How would we even begin to find them in this convulsion of earth and stone, and if we did, what could I do for them with the supplies in my medical case? Would I have to watch more of my friends die in this hellhole before we could get them to specialized medical aid on the surface? Then my wandering mind became more pragmatic: how do I get over, under, through, or around the next crushed area of the wall so I can find the next miner?

Dan and I walked into the level and up the wall, and found the second group of miners, about a half-dozen of them. The first sight was bone-chilling. One man had been instantly crushed to death by the Bump. The ones who were alive required medical help. Some had possible broken bones, others just needed their cuts bandaged. Soon Dan and I were separated, and I was on my own until the following day.

At the 13,800 level, the roof had collapsed and all we could see was rubble, except for a crawl space big enough to get to the bottom of the 13,800 wall. The wall itself was crushed and the packs demolished. The tremendous eruption from within the earth had forced the pavement clear into the roof. Anyone working that section of the wall had been instantly entombed. There was no question. I felt utterly helpless, knowing that their invisible bodies were only feet away.

The devastation was greatest at the middle of the wall. The pan line had been forced into the roof, and the working face had filled with coal. Whoever stood at the face with a pick in their hands at 8:06 PM had been buried in an avalanche as the coal face blasted towards them. Trickles of blood had run under the coal and compressed rubble, telling us where some of the men were. We marked those spots with chalk. Later the miners would know where to unearth the bodies.

It was an emotional shock, and I told myself, "My God, we've got to get to anyone who's alive!" I couldn't afford to dwell on the tragedies. A sense of urgency soon forced me over the rubble. Before long I was covered with dirt and sweat, and my muscles were tense. There I was, dragging the same medical bag I had brought into the No. 4 Mine Explosion. Some of the men had been lucky; they had been standing in the right places. Instead of being crushed, they had been forced into the air by the impact from below and the enormous compression of air that blasted them when the earth filled up the empty spaces.

Many of them only suffered minor injuries, such as sore arms and legs, or some had fractures. The rescuers took these men up to the surface.

By moving through the small spaces and in areas where the roof was unsupported, I was able to get to the bottom of the 13,400 wall. These unsupported areas were still seeping dust, which signalled the possibility of further shifting. This medical mission was not without danger. The first thing I noticed was that the 13,400 level had been filled completely near the wall. Nor could I get far up the 13,400 wall; the roof and pavement were crushed together again. Rubble and gas closed off access to the 13,000 and 12,600 levels.

Instead of shiny black coal faces on the walls separating the levels, I found metal pans, pack-wood sticks, timber, booms— and more blood. Lunch pails set back from the face told me that their owners were close by, yet invisible in the black mounds.

After treating some miners, I came to a group of rescuers. There, in the middle, was a man buried in coal. All I could see was the top of his left shoulder and a profile of his face. The left side of his head and ear were buried in hard-packed coal. It was Leon Melanson. His was the blackest face I'd seen. He moaned in agony. I approached and asked him, "Where does it hurt the most?"

"Everywhere," he said, with difficulty. "I'm being squeezed and I'm being crushed at the same time."

I opened my medical case, grabbed an ampoule of Demerol, and shot one hundred milligrams into his shoulder—the only exposed part of his body that would accept the needle. That was all I could do for him at that time. I knew that the others would continue digging him out, and so I moved on up the wall. The only way to keep going was to move out into the waste area. I was afraid the roof could come in there, but didn't have any choice.

When I had worked in the mines during the summers I had never been down the back slope of the No. 2 mine. I was crawling with barefaced men, and as we progressed up the 13,800 wall, I remarked that it seemed a long way to the next level. One of them told me that we were on the 13,400 wall and had crossed the level. I had been crawling through this rubble for four hours looking for something I had passed long ago! Not recognizing a level gives an idea of the extensive damage. The level runs at right angles to the walls. There are rails, heavy packs, heavy wooden or metal booms, and air lines. But here it just looked like another damaged section of the long wall of the mine.

Later, word was sent up the wall to me: "They want you back down with Leon Melanson because they want you to cut off a leg."

"What do you mean, 'cut off a leg?'"

"There's a dead man trapped with Leon and the dead man's leg is up under Leon's armpit, crossing his body. They can't get Leon out 'til they get that leg out of the way." It was four hours since I had left him.

So I went back down to Leon. On the way, I found a smashed miner's lamp. I cut the cord, about four feet long, and brought it with me in case I'd need to tie a tourniquet.[7] The miners had completely exposed his head and shoulders by that time, and you could see as far down as his waist. A leg came up, and the boot was jammed under Leon's armpit. The effect of the Demerol had worn off, so I gave him another shot in the shoulder straightaway.

He was still fully buried from the waist down, so his legs weren't visible. Having seen people trapped in bombed buildings overseas, something told me that this could be Leon's leg, and not that of his buddy who was completely buried behind and underneath him. When I refused, the rescue workers laughed at my explanation. All I could say back was, "Just keep on digging." This was heartbreaking work, chipping away at hard-packed coal with a live body underneath. They pitched in again. When Leon was finally dug out, his own broken and crushed leg was twisted up in front of him. Later, up at the local hospital, we tried to save that leg. It was finally amputated in Halifax. Leon also suffered internal damage from his hellish three-quarter burial.

By this time the rescuers had travelled up the walls as far as possible—crawling around, over, and under packs, rubble, fallen coal, stone, you name it. They were sure that no one else was alive in the accessible areas of the walls. Anyone who wasn't exposed at the time of the Bump had been killed instantly.

Much later, we heard that three men were trapped on the 13,400 level. We were about to witness a living nightmare. The roof and the floor had compressed together, leaving about a foot and a half clearance at the top. The three men were on the other side of this convulsed section of the level. Some machinery had been driven to the roof, and the draegermen couldn't clear it with the breathing packs on their backs. It was a job for barefaced men, if they could endure the gas. The trapped men would be ok as long as they stayed low. We didn't want to encourage them to try to go up over the machine in their weakened condition. Three times we were driven back down by the gas, but it seemed to be getting lighter. While waiting for our next attempt a chocolate bar caught my eye. It was sticking out of the shirt pocket of one of the barefaced rescuers. That made me realize how hungry and thirsty I was, and looking at my watch, I counted almost fourteen hours since I had eaten or had a drink of water.

"When did you eat last?" I asked the fellow.

"Oh, I had my breakfast an hour or so ago, before I came to the mines."

"Well, if you don't mind, I haven't had anything to eat since supper yesterday. How about that bar?"

So he handed it to me. They don't make chocolate bars that delicious nowadays. I began to wonder about those trapped men who had starved for four-and-a-half days after the Explosion.

Finally the gas diminished so that one fellow was able to get up over the machine. He started to help the others up. Since I was the smallest, I got up onto the machine, which was about five-feet across and began to pull one of the partially gassed trapped miners up towards me. He was "out of it" to the point of not knowing what he was doing; he braced one foot up into the roof while madly kicking the other. I couldn't pull him any further. I asked for my medical bag, injected a tranquilizer into his arm, and soon we were all in trouble. He relaxed all right, and so did his bowels. The poor fellows pulling on his legs said it was worse than mine gas. Once we got all that sorted out, the others came up over the machine much more cooperatively. One of the barefaced men told me that no other accessible areas remained; collapsed roofs and falls had closed off the unexplored areas.

Out of 174 men who were in the mine at the time of the Bump, 81 had made it to the surface by the following morning. But 19 of them were quite severely injured with broken bones and/or damage to internal organs. I wound up treating most if not all of these men at All Saints Hospital.

Some of the injured men recounted what happened to them from the time of the Bump until they were taken to the surface. When Clyde Murray Jr. came to, he was pinned to the roof. A prop was pressing against his chest, and coal and stone had piled under him. He thought the air was reversed and this worried him. Rescue workers sawed the prop, got him onto a stretcher, and moved him out. The Bump fired Sandy Wilson across a trip into a loader. The whole trip of twenty-six boxes was thrown to the low side. His light was blown off his hat. The two lights he could see belonged to Jack Scott and Ken Gilbert. Jack's legs were buried in a pile of coal and timber, and a big tool box had pinned Ken against the loader next to him. The level was closed off except for a space about a foot high.

Once the dust from the Bump cleared, George Hayden was buried up to his neck, but was able to dig himself out even though his leg was broken. Fred Hahnen relates that he and several other miners were preparing to shift the pan line, with their backs to the coal face, when the Bump hit. It threw them forward. The coal came down, caught their feet, and buried them. He was able to free his face and mouth and then had to wait until Buddy Rector and Russell MacLellan came along to free his chest and legs. The men said that their lights were knocked off their hats, but even after putting them back on they still couldn't see because of the density of dust and gases in the air.

By the time four o'clock in the morning rolled around, seventy-five of the survivors were on the surface. The newscasts were pessimistic about ever seeing the ninety-two who remained. As the miners continued to dig through the rubble, I went back up. It was eleven o'clock in the morning and I had been down there since nine o'clock the night before. I turned in my lamp, and a Salvation Army officer handed me a blessed cup of coffee, and then I disappeared into the multitude to find Helen. We went home and cooked up a sizeable breakfast, which was followed by a hot bath and bed. After being awake for over thirty hours, it didn't take me long to conk out.

At the time of the Bump, the walls on the three levels were in line. According to the mining experts, this system was the safest, though it had been hotly contested by the old miners of Springhill. After the Bump, they still stuck to their own theory.

The first day, we had heard nothing positive from the news media. "There is no possible hope of getting anyone out alive," they drummed into their radio and newspaper audiences.

But the old miners knew better. They said, "We've got live people from the top and bottom of the walls on the 13,400 level. There's bound to be live men from the same sections of the walls up above. And we've got to get to them." The more pessimistic the media reports became, the more vigorously they contested them.

Families whose relations had been working on the middle of the walls were a lot less hopeful. Even then, most stuck to the miner's watchword: the men are alive until we find their bodies. And then there were some who had given up hope to the point of digging graves. Soon, two and three funerals a day cast a pall over the town.

Springhillers baked hams, breads, and cookies for their neighbours and friends who had been stricken, not knowing if their relations were alive or dead. There were always friends in the house; nobody was left alone. Sometimes the townspeople would just sit there without saying anything, just to be there in case anything was needed. We took it for granted; this is how it had always been. But for people from away, such camaraderie was something new.

By the morning of October 24, 1958, it was clear that any further survivors would be down there for some time. Clearing the rock falls and collapsed levels was tremendously time consuming. In some areas, the trolley rails, which normally had a ten- to twelve-foot clearance from the roof, had been pushed up flat against the roof. The debris had to be moved, yet there was no place to put it. And the new tunnels dug through the damaged areas had to be shored up by timbers, which were carried in by hand in the absence of trollies.

Meanwhile the surface was a hotbed of activity. The armouries had been prepared as a morgue. Two local restaurateurs were preparing meals for all who needed them—at no charge. After they ran out of food, they began using food sent in by the government. The Boy Scouts' tent advertised: WANT ANYTHING DONE ASK A BOY SCOUT. They washed dishes, carried food, peeled potatoes, served meals, looked after children, did housework, and just about anything else that was needed.

A bevy of ambulances congregated by the mine entrance: Lindsay Funeral Home, the navy, the Red Cross, and St. John Ambulance. The Halifax police were also present. Bagnell's Dry Cleaners had sent a panel truck from Halifax, as did other companies. The Red Cross wound up sending in over twenty thousand dollars worth of supplies of clothing and food. The Royal Canadian Legion and the Auxiliary were also there since many of the trapped men were veterans.

The Queen sent her concerns, as did ambassadors from many countries. A Toronto television station had already set up a nationwide fundraising appeal to assist the families in need.

By this time, the rescue effort included twenty draegermen from Springhill, twelve from Glace Bay, thirteen from Stellarton, thirteen from New Waterford, and over two hundred barefaced men.

Press coverage was massive. The office of the Canadian National Telegraph was busy around the clock. There 137 reporters covering the story wrote 110,000 words as they filed their news stories.

While some of the rescuers continued working to penetrate the levels, others laboured to recover bodies. This became more gruesome as the days progressed. It was warm in there, and the bodies that had been compressed by coal would balloon out as soon as they were uncovered. They stank from decomposition. Some of the miners reported that the corpses dripped on them once they were unearthed. It took extremely dedicated men to continue this work day after day, without the hope that live men might be found. But the miners were committed to account for every man, and that's what kept them going.

When a dead miner was found, he was taken up to the surface in an airtight coffin. To establish positive identity, a mine official, a miner's union official, and a doctor (myself in most cases) examined him. All three had to agree on the identity. If the man was unrecognizable, his identity was established by either the check number on his lamp or body marks such as an amputated index finger, scars, or false teeth. The dead miner's minister or priest was then notified. He, in turn, notified the family. The news media were the last to get the word.

Bodies that eluded these identity procedures were kept in the ambulance shed at the mine's entrance until the man's name could be determined.

At the 13,000 level, the miners realized it would be impossible to clear the immense deluge of fallen debris. So they started to "rib up the high-side coal," meaning they started to dig a new tunnel through the untouched coal on the high side of the level. They had 160 feet to go before reaching the foot of the 13,000 wall. At some point during their tunnelling efforts, my phone rang at home. This was five-and-a-half days after the Bump. I had just been filling out death certificates and recording the men's names, check numbers, and injuries in a mine official's notebook. In most cases for injuries I was listing "MSCC" for "Multiple Severe Contusions and Crushing"....

"Dr. Burden?"

"Yes?"

"Can you come out to the mine immediately? We've got more men alive!"

"Ok. Be right there."

With a rush of adrenaline I pushed my logbook in my pocket, grabbed my coat, and drove off. The mine manager, George Calder, was on the phone. As I walked in, he signalled for me to come over close. He was jotting down names and pointing to one with his left hand: CALEB RUSHTON. He knew Caleb had been married to my sister. By the time he was through, he had written down twelve names. Next to two of them he scrawled SEVERELY INJURED, and hung up the phone.

"Well, thank God some more of them are alive," he exclaimed. "But the rescue tunnel hasn't reached them yet." His excitement was contagious.

"We'll have to get to them," I replied.

"What are we going to need down there?" he asked. "We'll have to get them food and water."

The rescue group gathered the supplies we would need and then we headed underground to the 13,000 level. One of the teams of miners had come across a broken air line along the roof that led into the wall. This line was six inches in diameter, and as Blair Phillip was taking an air sample to test for gas, he heard a distant voice: "There are twelve of us here." It was Gorley Kempt! He had seen the flash of Blair's lamp through the pipe!

In his excitement, Blair yelled back, "Stay where you are. We'll come as quickly as possible." Since they had been trapped for five-and-a-half days without food or water, there wasn't much chance they'd be going anywhere! Along with Gorley were Harold Brine, Joseph Holloway, Wilfred Hunter, Larry Leadbetter, Levi Milley, Theodore Michniak, Caleb Rushton, Bowman Maddison, Eldred Lowther, Joseph MacDonald, and Hugh Guthro. We had no idea how far away they were from the break in the pipe.

NOTES

1. A nine-foot-high coal seam along the walls in between the levels: See diagram page 146.

2. Room and pillar system: When you cut out one block of coal, you leave the adjacent block of coal intact to support the roof.

3. Long wall retreating system: You mine towards the slope and let the roof fall into the empty space where the coal has been removed.

4. Travelling road: The safer walkway between two rows of packs, used to go up or down a wall.

5. Safety lamps: Lamps carried to detect mine gases.

6. Gas: Mostly methane.

7. Tourniquet: This cord is on display at the Miners' Museum in Springhill.

12. *More Rescues and the* Ed Sullivan Show

Among the supplies we brought with us were a fifty-foot copper pipe and a plastic hose. These would enable us to send water and soup through the pipe to the men. A doctor DOSCO had brought down from Cape Breton got it into his head that we should be mixing vitamins into the fluids. Captain Bruce Harcourt of the Salvation Army, who had prepared the nourishment, conveyed this message to me. I vehemently opposed the idea because the riboflavin and other vitamin components would make the men sick as soon as they smelled it. I asked the captain, "Have you ever sucked or bitten into a vitamin capsule?" So I resolved to check on all the fluids to be sent in, because I didn't want them nauseated and vomiting after their first sips of nourishment. I got my way and the vitamins went by the wayside.

The voices carried well through the pipe, but we were still guessing how far we'd have to tunnel to reach them. First we tried to push the fifty-foot length of half-inch copper pipe through; it didn't make it. So we pulled it back out, taped the plastic pipe to it, and sent that in. But it was snug and rather than risk plugging the pipe—our only means of getting food and water in—we pulled it out and sent up to the surface for a hundred-foot copper pipe.

When we pushed this through, it made it to where Gorley was, but he asked if it could come any further to reach the others. The air line was partially filled with coal dust, and now, with the smaller pipe inside, we couldn't see because the air was blowing the dust out our end and into our faces. We cut off the excess pipe at our end, and after measuring it, we realized we still had eighty-three feet of solid coal ahead of us. Others had sent to Amherst for a brand new five-gallon pressure pump—the type used for spraying trees—and we taped it to the end of the copper pipe. We sent in the first tank of water at 6:00 PM.

Up to that time the rescue miners had cut through about a dozen feet during each eight-hour shift. Once we knew there were live men on the other side, it only took fourteen hours to go the remaining eighty-three feet.

When the first water came through the other end, the men were caught off guard. It sprayed everywhere. They chastised us for wasting it! We assured them there was plenty more where that came from. Catching a trickle of water in a thin-mouthed water bottle in the pitch dark must have been some challenge, particularly in a weakened state. I instructed them to take one mouthful at a time, counting to five hundred in between. I came up with this number because I knew they would count fast.

At 6:15 PM we sent in two tankfuls of hot coffee with sugar and no milk. The sugar would provide quick nourishment and the caffeine, stimulation. I recorded all this in the mine official's book I had thrust into my pocket at home.

At 8:10 we sent a tankful of hot tomato soup. Gorley sounded good but he said that Ted Michniak and Joe MacDonald needed help. George Scott, one of the rescuers, had been talking to the trapped men in his broad Scots accent and Gorley replied: "Take the marbles out of your mouth and speak English." It was heartening to see he hadn't lost his sense of humour. At 8:25 we sent another tankful of soup through the pipe. The trapped men asked how much further we had to go before reaching them. We didn't want them to know, so we said, "About ten feet or more."

"Ok. We'll lay down and rest."

The tunnel we were digging was small. If I sat down I took up all the room, which might have measured three feet by three feet. We didn't have proper roof supports. As the mine continued to have small bumps, the dust and small chunks of coal would fall from the roof onto our legs. We were pretty sure there wouldn't be another big bump, but we knew the roof could cave in around us at any time. One miner would dig at the "face" of the tunnel, on his knees, with a pick whose handle had been cut short. Another miner would pull the coal from between his legs, while someone else would scoop it into buckets with a short-handled shovel. The buckets were then passed back to the men who were sitting side to side along the tunnel wall. The last fellow in the bucket brigade finally got rid of the coal at the other end. The miners took turns at the backbreaking work with the pick. Considering their progress that last eighty-three feet, you have to marvel at their unflagging effort. Especially when you consider the poor air they were breathing; manual labour is much more strenuous when there's less oxygen in the blood supply.

Someone suggested I take a break from the bucket line, so I moved out of the line of fire, leaving my medical case behind. Suddenly I smelled rum and yelled: "John, put that back." It was good for a laugh, because I knew who had grabbed hold of the rum bottle without even seeing him.

I felt a slight movement of air in the tunnel at 8:38, and noted it in my book. Before this, it had been dead. The pace of work picked up. At 9:55 the trapped men requested more water and we sent in another tankful. By 11:00 the voices seemed to be weaker, but they claimed they could hear digging close by. At 12:30, George Calder, the mine manager, called to them, and Harold Bryan answered in a strong voice. We fed them more water. At 1:10 AM, Levi Milley's voice rang out loud and clear: "We can hear digging behind a pack."

At 2:25 AM on that Thursday, October 30, we broke through. "We're through!" resounded through the level. A blast of air and dust filled the tunnel, and after some minutes we could see. At that time I was still eighty-five feet back, looking after the refreshments at our end of the pipe.

Some of the trapped men were standing, others sat on the mine floor pavement.[1] They seemed to be in fair condition. A few of the miners and I kept going and crawled through a small opening underneath a large, loose stone that was precariously balanced. The two injured men were on the other side. Joe MacDonald was sitting with his back propped against a conveyor pan that had tilted on edge. His legs were straight out in front. I could see that his upper leg was fractured, and the bone was sticking out through the skin.

"How's your leg?" I asked.

"Awful sore," he said in a pained voice.

I gave him one-hundred milligrams of Demerol and went over about twenty feet to Teddie Michniak. He was leaning against a pile of coal with a face so black I couldn't see his expression. I noticed the two of them were shielding their eyes from the lights so I covered mine with a handkerchief.

Teddie said, "Thanks. Glad you got here," in a weary voice. I was the first to reach him. He was holding his damaged arm against his chest. I felt his shoulder. His arm was dislocated from the socket. I took his pulse as a matter of course. All I could do was make sure he was fit to be moved. I went back and forth between the two of them until the miners had that rock stabilized. Ironically, someone found a lunch pail full of mouldy food behind a pack! So close yet so far away, and in the dark. The stretchers came in, we loaded them on, and they were carried out of their prison. I made sure they had handkerchiefs over their eyes and told the miners how important this would be at the surface. Considering how weak the other ten were, they went up on stretchers as well. At 4:20 AM I scribbled "Last Man Out," and with my aching muscles part crawled and part walked out of the black hole.

The trapped men told harrowing stories. The Bump knocked Gorley's lamp off and all he could hear was Caleb hollering. By the time Gorley had recovered his lamp and gotten to Caleb, Levi had unburied him. All twelve frantically tried to get up the wall, but couldn't. So they went in the opposite direction, tunnelling through three stone walls before coming to a large fall. They couldn't get around it, even by going into the waste. They found some lunchboxes and water cans that were crushed and useless, except for one gallon of water, which ended up lasting them five days. Using a cap from an aspirin bottle, they each took one capful of water at a time so as to share it evenly. While we were tunnelling towards them, they worried that we were digging in the wrong direction, so misled were they by the vibrations they heard.

Finding them proved that men could still be alive at the top of a wall, so the miners' efforts redoubled to get to the next wall up. This was the last bastion of safety for any more possibly trapped men.

Meanwhile, aluminum coffins continued to ascend. Seventy-four were brought up, in all; the seventy-fifth man was to die in hospital two weeks afterwards. He was the only one to die on the surface from injuries caused by the Bump.

The rescued miners got a great lift when His Royal Highness Prince Philip visited on October 31. He had attended a meeting in Ottawa, and directed that his jet be brought down in the Moncton airport. It was about 5:15 PM. Nova Scotia Premier Robert Stanfield, the Honourable George C. Nowlan, Minister of National Revenue, and the Honourable Stephen Pyke, Minister of Labour and Public Works were there to greet him. They headed straight for Springhill and Mayor Gilroy met the Prince at All Saints Hospital. They went through the wards and the Prince spoke to each man and shook their hands. He also visited the less severe casualties in the emergency hospital that had been set up in the armouries.

His last stop was the mine site before returning to the plane. I was introduced to him, but he was more interested in the rescued miners. This was the first time I had been in contact with royalty since the war; it was a nice feeling to shake his hand.

Arnold Patterson, public relations officer for the coal company, phoned. Ed Sullivan wanted some of the trapped miners on his show that Sunday evening and Arnie wanted Helen and myself to go along. Talk about a contrast from what we'd been doing down in the mine! It would be the three of us, plus Phyllis Griffiths, a reporter with the *Toronto Telegram*, Gorley Kempt and his wife Margie, and Caleb Rushton and his wife Pat. I was chosen because I could represent the rescuers and also look after Gorley and Caleb's medical needs.

It was the second anniversary of the Explosion—November 1. As I was pulling clothing out of the closet, the phone rang again.

"Can you come? There's more men alive in the mine!" shocked me down into my shoes. Afterwards someone said, "He fell out of bed and into the mine." The call came in at 4:45 AM and at 5:00 I was at the pit. At 5:12, I went down on a trolley with a group of barefaced men.

I was crawling by the intersection of the wall and the 13,000 level, wondering how many more are there, and how badly are they hurt? Then I saw a hole just big enough to squeeze through—about two feet around. I stuck my head in and saw John Calder and Bennie Roy.

"Who do you have?" I asked.

John said, "We think it's Barney Martin. He's in a small open space. We still have to shift more stone to get to him." So I waited twenty minutes or so, lying on my belly in the rubble. After they cleared the way, they supported the roof, and by 6:20 we got to Barney. I saw him feet first as they were pushing him through the opening. A few barefaced men and I gently pulled until we had him out. His body had been stressed by sitting in such a tight position with his legs forced up. He was barely breathing but his eyes were wide open. His sounds were unintelligible, his mouth likely full of coal dust. We put him on a stretcher and poured a few mouthfuls of coffee down his throat. He was in a semi-coma and severely dehydrated. No use checking for internal damages until we get him up to the surface, I thought, and away he went.

Meanwhile, John and Bennie moved forward and two more rescuers climbed in to join them. I followed and we all moved farther up the wall. John and Bennie were the first to see the group of men standing in an open space alongside the level.

"How many are here?" he asked.

"Give me some water and I'll sing you a song," Maurice Ruddick replied. Maurice was known as the singing miner; later some of his family members were to become professional singers.

I handed them the water can and they passed it around. Besides Maurice, there were Douglas Jewkes, Herb Pepperdine, Garnet Clarke, Currie Smith, and Frank Hunter. They all seemed to be in fair shape. And then I saw Percy Rector's body, limply hanging from a pack. His arm had been caught and crushed by the pack. The men told us he had lived until Tuesday night. They also said that since they hadn't heard any rapping on the pipes they figured there was no one else alive on that wall. The rescue team included a mine inspector, an engineer, a general manager, and an overman—a lot of top brass. As soon as our lights entered the area, one of the trapped men became extremely agitated. It was the sight of his dead buddy. He said, "If that body isn't covered, I'm going to go out of my mind."

At 7:10 we fed them hot chocolate, and at 7:20 tomato soup. daylight saving time had changed back to standard time while they had been trapped, and they had somehow set their watches to the correct time. We found this out when they asked us the time, which synchronized with theirs.

Maurice Ruddick was particularly glad to see us. John Calder addressed him: "Maurice, the Workmen's Compensation Board sent me down here specifically to get you out."

Puzzled, Maurice asked, "Why?"

"They said if we don't find you, they'll have to pay so much for your wife and twelve children that there won't be enough for the others."

On the previous Monday, they celebrated Garnet Clarke's twenty-ninth birthday by dividing one sandwich into seven sections—followed by one capful of water each to wash it down. Their water lasted until the following day; from then on they chewed on anything that would produce saliva. Bark from a pit prop and coal were handiest.

At 7:30 we fed them some more tomato soup and at 8:15 they started down the wall. Rescuers supported them as they stumbled half from weakness and half from tripping on the rubble. We reached an area where the roof had fallen in, so we helped the men over the fall and down to the level before putting them onto stretchers. I told one of the rescuing miners, "I'm going to report you!"

He said, "Huh?"

"No qualified miner would work in a place without roof supports."

By 8:45 I was on the trolley with them, headed for the surface.

At the beginning of their ordeal, these men had had to make a tough decision. There was Percy Rector's arm, caught in a pack. If they tried to amputate it, they figured he could die from shock or loss of blood. So they chose to leave him be, hoping rescuers would come in time. We were four days too late.

I got home at 10:00 PM and had to get ready to leave for the Moncton airport at 5:00 the next morning. I only had a small amount of cash in my pocket and these were the days before automatic teller machines or credit cards. There were only a couple of exposures left on the film in the camera, and there was no more film. So I resigned myself to being unprepared for this whirlwind trip to New York, and we retired well after midnight. The next day got off to a good start on the plane when one of the reporters flying out of Springhill gave me a few extra rolls of thirty-five millimetre film.

Lord Beaverbrook was on our flight from Saint John, New Brunswick to Boston and we were all introduced. The pilot, Captain Muir, told us we were flying at the height above ground that the men had been trapped below ground—about three miles.

At the Boston airport, Arnie took us into a throng of journalists, photographers, and TV cameramen. Dozens of reporters were stumbling over one another to talk to the trapped men. We held up the plane because they wouldn't let us go, and then we finally managed to escape.

The plane was packed, and on the way in to New York City it hit me, what lay ahead of us. In a very short time Caleb, Gorley, and I would be televised internationally on the most popular network show. Millions of people would be watching. And this would be within twenty-four hours of crawling through rubble a mile underground in a convulsed mine rescue, where the light was so poor I could see no more than six people at a time.

For Caleb and Gorley the contrast would even be more phenomenal. They had only been out of the mine a couple of days after having been trapped in that hellhole for five-and-a-half days without food, water, or light. I had only gotten two hours sleep in the proceeding thirty-six hours. It was a battle between exhaustion and excitement, and that's how I flew into the big city. The six of us were about to become faces in an international news story.

On the way to the Park Sheraton Hotel our taxi drove past the Trans-lux Theater at West 49th Street and Broadway. The entire front of the marquee was devoted to these words: MORE MEN ALIVE. It was a news theatre, and suddenly we felt right at home in downtown New York City.

Photographers dogged us during our entire visit. Some were just plain jerks, asking us to look up at the tall buildings, as if we were country hicks who had never seen buildings before. I told them to go to hell.

We arrived at the hotel at 1:30 in the afternoon and there was only one thing on my mind as we checked in: a steak dinner. It wasn't long before I was cutting into a great big sirloin, thanks to room service.

Since we were such a big party we always took two taxis; invariably, I ended up paying for one of them. The little bit of cash I had with me was rapidly running through my fingers.

At 3:30 we were escorted into the CBS television studio for more photographs and interviews—and to meet Ed Sullivan. Some of the photographers asked us to get up on stage. We obliged, and then they vanished when Ed Sullivan appeared. Gorley, Caleb, and I were stranded there on stage, so we moved back against the curtain to make ourselves inconspicuous. Ed walked to the mike with a stately gait and welcomed the audience to the afternoon show. In an instant, he took command. Then he spotted us and turned the mike over to someone else. He strode over and said, very directly, "Well, who are you?" We must have looked like the Three Stooges.

I said, "These are the trapped men from Springhill."

Suddenly he was very friendly. We all shook hands and he said, "I'm very pleased to have you here on the show." I explained that the newsmen had set us up on the stage. Then he noticed how pale and weak Gorley was.

"Just stay here for a moment," he said and went to get a chair for Gorley. This was both compassionate and practical (I'm sure he didn't want anyone collapsing onstage). Then he introduced each of us to the audience, and we stayed up there for the rest of the rehearsal.

Ed told the audience this show was to commemorate the heroism of the individual, and he motioned towards us, and the heroism of the small nation of Israel. He introduced some Israeli talent and then the Mormon Tabernacle Choir.

Afterwards, on the way back to the hotel, we saw the front page newspaper headlines announcing the rescue of the last seven men from the mines at home. We came back to the CBS studio in time for the televised show at 7:30. Caleb, Gorley, and I were seated in row four in the centre, with our wives right in front of us. We didn't go onstage during the actual show partly because of the length of the show and partly because the rescued miners were feeling weak. But Ed asked us to stand partway through. He introduced us to everyone who had tuned in across the continent. Then he made an appeal for funds by mentioning the Springhill Miners' Disaster Fund.

After the show we met him again, and I showed him the notes I had made in the mine official's book. He autographed it, inscribing: "Billy—We are just as proud of your father as all of Canada. Sincerely, Ed Sullivan." Then he handed me his own personal cheque for one thousand dollars made out to the Miners' Disaster Fund. By mentioning the fund on the air he raised a great deal of money, and the fund eventually collected two million dollars. The press continued to hound us afterwards, and we were still getting telephone calls in our rooms at 2:30 AM. At that point I told the hotel clerk to relay the messages to me so Caleb and Gorley could get some rest.

The next day we had some time for sightseeing. As we got into the cab in the morning, the driver said, "Aren't you the people from the mines in Nova Scotia?" Between the Ed Sullivan Show and the newspapers, I guess our faces had been spread around pretty good by then. We had become celebrities overnight! The next day, November 4, we left our once-in-a-lifetime extravaganza and headed back to good old Springhill.

The last bodies were being recovered from the mine and identified, while the town cemetery was being expanded. But the identification procedures lapsed while I was away. One body was identified by the man's sister and two friends when other methods failed. Instead of holding it for further corroboration by a doctor and a mine official, it was taken directly to the man's home for burial. I returned from New York exhausted, but was called to the mine when the body of this previously "identified" man was discovered. I had to go to the man's home, explain the mix-up to his wife, and arrange for the exchange of bodies. The funeral of the first man was scheduled for that afternoon. This was the only case of misidentification, and from then on we adhered to our original system.

At that time twenty-two miners were killed in a mine in Bishop, Virginia, and the Town of Springhill sent our sympathies.

When the nineteen trapped men had convalesced, they held a small party for just themselves and their wives. Joe MacDonald was the last to be released from hospital, and the party was at his house. I was honoured to be the only one invited outside that group. Some of the men had been trapped in both disasters. It was a joyous time with everyone celebrating something that most of us take for granted: being alive.

Next, the Governor of Georgia invited the rescued miners and their families to come recuperate in his sunny southern climate. Maurice Ruddick was of mixed-race and the State of Georgia's segregation laws caused some problems. Some of the others said they wouldn't go without him, and then he said he would go, accepting the fact that he would be separated from the group. He felt everyone would benefit from the invitation. On November 18, forty-four Springhillers set out on an all-expenses-paid trip to Georgia, and came back two weeks later with all kinds of stories that kept the town buzzing for days.

Back home, the news wasn't so sunny. Whereas approximately one thousand men had been working in the mines before the disaster, about nine hundred were now jobless. And the final word had come from Sir Roy Dobson, head of Avro, which was DOSCO's parent company: the No. 2 mine was too dangerous to operate. Its future was sealed. Efforts to reopen the No. 4 mine also crashed into a dead end.

Meanwhile, back in Hamilton, Ontario, an honour was bestowed on us. The Royal Humane Association Gold Medal, Canada's highest recognition for bravery in life-saving, was designated for Springhill. The medal had never been awarded to a group before. Three-quarters of a year later, on August 8, 1959, it was presented and a dedication ceremony was held at the Cumberland Railway and Coal Company Park in Springhill and I was a platform guest. In a separate ceremony, five rescuers, who were also scoutmasters with the Boy Scouts, were awarded Scout Silver Crosses in Ottawa.

Attracting new industry to the town became a desperately high priority. A citizens' advisory committee was established to tackle this. On May 28, 1959, the federal government announced that a prison farm would be built here as a rehabilitation project. As of 1991, approximately three hundred people are employed in the medium-security prison that holds about five hundred inmates.

William Stevenson, one of the miners rescued the first night after the Bump, died in All Saints Hospital on November 24, 1958, bringing the total number killed to seventy-five.

Maurice Ruddick, the miner who offered to trade a song for a drink of water, was named Citizen of the Year for 1958, a Canada-wide honour. He went to Toronto to receive a bronze plaque on February 15, 1959, and was also introduced from the floor of the Ontario Legislature.

The crowning moment came when the Carnegie Hero Fund Commission presented a special gold medal and a bronze plaque to the rescuers. The citation on the plaque reads:

Resolved, that the Carnegie Hero Fund Commission award a gold medal to the officials and workmen of the Dominion Steel and Coal Corporation, Limited, and local doctors who risked their lives attempting to rescue one hundred and seventy-four miners who were trapped by an underground convulsion in a company mine at Springhill, Nova Scotia, on October 23, 1958.

I remembered the leaves I had spent in Dunfermline during the war, and especially the museum Andrew Carnegie had endowed. It felt like a small world indeed when I saw in my mind's eye the fossilized tree trunk from Joggins, Cumberland County, that had been displayed in front of that museum in the town where Andrew Carnegie was born.

Springhillers weren't too crazy about the decision to keep this medal in the public archives in Halifax. But a copy was made for display in the federal building in Springhill, and then the original medal was moved to Springhill in 1988. It now resides in the town hall, and the replica is on display at the Miners' Museum. At a ceremony in Springhill's Capitol Theatre, Premier Stanfield presented Monson Harrison, president of the United Mine Workers of America, with a blue ribbon which bore a gold stamp of the medal, on behalf of all of the heroes. Each of us was then given an identical blue ribbon.

The National Research Council of the National Academy of Sciences in Washington, DC, funded their thirteenth disaster study, entitled: *Individual and Group Behaviour in a Coal Mine Disaster*. Sociologists, psychologists, and psychiatrists from Dalhousie University in Halifax and Acadia University in Wolfville carried out the research. I provided information that was requested of me, and was acknowledged as follows: "R. A. Burden…contributed invaluable assistance as a special medical and technical consultant," in the book that was published in 1960.

Books and magazine articles abounded, many with inaccuracies. Yet many stories remain untold and are vanishing into oblivion. Over thirty years have passed. The people who were involved, and the memories of others, are fading away.

The final casualty of the Springhill mines occurred some time after the Bump. Bootleg mines sprang up as miners worked illegally to get coal to heat their homes. One of these mines had tunnelled into the workings of the old Syndicate Mine, which had been sealed for many years.

A legal company was formed to take out the pillars of coal close to the surface. Again, I entered the mine in an emergency this time to investigate a sudden death.

I walked down the slope until I saw him leaning against a 22,000 volt transformer. He had slipped and fallen. One of his fingers had jammed into a small opening in the box, and electrocution was instant. What a fate—of all places for his fingers to land.

There were just two tiny marks on him: one burn on his finger and the other on the bottom of his foot where the current had jumped through a hole in his rubber boot to the wet mine floor.

No rescue this time, but another death claimed by the mines of Springhill. The coal was subsequently removed, and then the mine was sealed off past a depth of two hundred feet. It was converted to the Miners' Museum, where visitors can go today to dig a bit of souvenir coal from these historic coal fields.

NOTES

1. Pavement: The stone floor in a mine.

13. Wringing Urine from Diapers and Other Rewards

THE TOWN WAS IN SHOCK. IF THE EXPLOSION, THE FIRE, AND NOW THE BUMP HAD HAPPENED TO A PERSON'S BODY WITHIN A three year period, two legs and an arm would be missing, and that person would be severely traumatized. A heart, a brain, and one leg would remain. Perhaps the biggest loss we suffered over time was, in a certain sense, the heart of the town: the young people moved away since we had virtually no jobs to offer them. This robbed us of much of our future. Beautiful homes were being sold for peanuts...a few thousand dollars...as people moved out west.

But I don't want to paint too bleak a picture. During the last disaster, Mayor Gilroy remarked: "There will always be a Springhill." Although coal was the soul of the town for many years, today it's gone. The only mine is at the Miners' Museum, where tourists can go a couple hundred feet down to pick souvenir coal to take home with them. Springhill has become a tourist destination, not only because of its mining legacy, but also on account of the renowned singer Anne Murray, who was born and raised here. In recent years, music lovers have come from afar to tour the beautiful Anne Murray Centre, where her gold and platinum records are displayed along with a rich array of memorabilia. New industries gradually came to Springhill and we began to develop a new economic base. The character of the town is different because of this. The coal that used to flow through the system of every Springhiller, from boyhood and girlhood, has become a thing of the past. Light manufacturing has begun to spring up in the new industrial parks.

Tough economic times also have a way of getting people closer together. This was certainly the case with St. Andrew's Presbyterian United Church and the Wesley United Church. They couldn't continue independently so they united in the strictest sense of the word.

I had joined the Rotary Club that first summer back in Springhill, was vice-president during the Bump, and became president the next year. Rotarians from all over the world sent money to the Disaster Relief Fund, which had been established after the 1956 Explosion. One of our major projects was the Crippled Children's Clinic which was held twice a year in Springhill. "Crippled" referred to any disabilities that would stop the child's vocational development. These included lung problems, speech impediments, asthma, heart condition, arthritis, severe burns, and eyesight disorders. Five specialists from Halifax came up to treat between two and three hundred children from different sections of the county. We even brought in a speech therapist from Scotland. Once a year some of the children spent two weeks in speech therapy in the Carlton Hotel in Springhill, and the Rotary Club picked up the tab.

Whipper Billy Watson, the professional wrestler, had been visiting the larger cities across Canada to promote the Crippled Children's Clinics. When Herb Zorychta was still president of our Rotary Club, he extended an invitation to Whipper Billy. He said he'd be willing to visit any town that had a "Timmie," which was any crippled child who would represent the group for a year. He was slated to return to Toronto for a wrestling match that Sunday night, but he cancelled and came to Springhill instead. He wouldn't let us reimburse him, saying, "I always pay my way on the trips across Canada. That's my donation to the cause."

Mayor Ralph Gilroy and Whipper Billy Watson toughed it out in a mock wrestling match at the Capitol Theatre. The Whipper was taken from the mines, to the hospital, to the schools, and by the end of the day he had rubbed shoulders with most of the town. The success of his visit showed up the following year when twice as many donations to the Crippled Children's Fund came in, in spite of the disasters. After our visit, he began visiting other smaller towns around the country. The Crippled Children Society certainly owes a great deal to this benefactor.

After twenty years with the Rotary Club, I sent in my resignation; the time constraints of the medical office, the hospital, and the prison were taking their toll. They sent back a surprise letter making me an honourary member instead. I've enjoyed my affiliation with the organization over the years. In 1959 there was a Rotary meeting in San Francisco at the same time an annual meeting was held at the United Nations in New York. More people from more countries attended our meeting, and I gained a new appreciation for the true international scope of the Rotary Club.

After our third son, David, was born in 1958, we tried to get a housekeeper since Helen had her hands full just looking after the kids. In a town where money was so scarce after the disasters, we didn't expect to have any trouble. As it turned out, people were either moving away or they were on welfare. The ones on welfare were afraid they would be cut off if they did any work. We couldn't get anyone, and Helen had to look after my medical phone calls, take care of the children, *and* do the housework.

It got even worse after Tim was born. But when it came to babysitting, we were blessed. Anne Murray, who was a teenager at that time, would come and look after the three boys: the infant, David, five-year-old Kent, and seven-year-old Bill. And she never accepted any money. The Hammond chord organ in our living room was payment enough. Once the kids were asleep, she would sit and play to her heart's content. Anne had been studying piano with our neighbour, Mrs. Gladys Matthews, and was already on her way to an extraordinary career.

Our fourth son, Tim, was born in 1960, after Helen had made several trips to hospital. Two years later at our cottage in Heather Beach, we were all sitting down to supper. Tim was in a highchair, flanked by the other kids on both sides. Helen had just set down a large glass of milk in front of each of them. All of a sudden, Tim downed his and then reached across to his brothers' glasses and downed two more in nothing flat. I knew something was wrong, so I brought him into the washroom and checked his urine. This was easy to do with the Clinitest tablets I had on hand. I dropped a tablet in and waited for the colour to change. It went from greenish to yellowish to bright orange to a dark brown. Which meant diabetes.

This was going to be a major problem for both Helen and myself, not to mention for Tim. He had to be put on insulin right away; Helen and I had to administer it daily until he was able to take over for himself at age twelve. And we had to test his urine regularly. Since he was still in diapers, there was only one way: to wring them out. Need I say more? It was a shock knowing that Tim would have this for the rest of his life, and that we would have to watch for complications. We had to serve him substitute foods, but this didn't seem so bad because we'd say, "You must be somebody special because you're getting this stuff and the other kids aren't."

The kids were always active and inquisitive, and took an interest in everything around them. They plowed through books, got involved in sports, fought with each other, and protected one another from either the other siblings or the neighbours. Come to think of it, they weren't too different from Audrey and me!

One unusual medical call came just minutes after Dr. Carson Murray suffered a severe attack of kidney stones and was rushed to Halifax. That left Dr. Fisher and myself. The call came in from Athol Road, and I went out to examine a young girl with acute appendicitis. Her condition was obvious after asking some questions and feeling her abdomen. Something had to be done right away, so I brought her to hospital. Dr. Fisher gave her the anaesthetic and I removed the appendix, which had become very inflamed; any longer, and it would have ruptured. It was one of those cases when everything went perfectly, and only took twenty minutes from start to finish. This was the first time I performed an inter-abdominal surgery with no assistant—and it certainly wasn't the last.

The Cumberland branch of the Nova Scotia Medical Society elected me to the board of Maritime Medical Care (MMC), a private insurance company that predated medicare. I served on the board for fourteen years. MMC was a member of the Western Conference of Pre-Paid Medical Service Plans of North America. I guess we qualified since we were west of Newfoundland. When MSI came onstream, the provincial government chose MMC to administer it. During my term, the board was responsible for a broad spectrum of the medical services of the province. I was appointed to the executive for eleven years, and served as vice-president for two years and president for two years. While I was president, I also served as an observer for the Nova Scotia Health Services Commission, which oversees MSI.

In 1989, the government of Great Britain issued the Normandy Medal to all those who served in the invasion of Normandy and during the few weeks after D-Day, and I was honoured to receive one. During this time of recognition, the president of the International Mine Workers of America presented me with a plaque for my work during the mine disasters in a ceremony on Miners' Memorial Day in Springhill.

Still another thrill was receiving the Baden-Powell badge. The local Boy Scout troop presented it to me at a banquet for my contribution as president of the Springhill Scout district, and also for my overall help with the troop, which distinguished itself by earning six Queen's Scouts Awards in two years.

Further accolades came when the Rotary Club named me a Paul Harris Fellow, the Legion gave me the Diamond Jubilee Medal and a forty-five year pin, and then the Medical Society of Nova Scotia made me a senior member in 1987. Then, in 1991, I was made senior member of the Canadian Medical Association. Perhaps these are just rewards for getting old.

For the past twenty-five years I have been the medical officer at the medium-security all-men's prison, which is one of the biggest prisons in Canada. The first day it opened we received 30 men, and then it was 30 a month until we had about 400. Since then we've had as many as 550 at a time. I treat a variety of injuries, including broken bones, appendectomies, burns, knife wounds—just about everything, but no maternities! I'm either on call seven days a week, twenty-four hours a day, or I'm responsible for a qualified doctor who is.

At the moment I'm chief of staff of the Springhill Hospital, chairman of the Accreditation Committee, I'm on the executive of the medical staff, trustee of the board of the hospital, and serve on the hospital's Building Committee. In the good old days I served on twenty-three committees at once, which meant three 3-hour meetings every two weeks, on average, which I can't say I miss.

About eighteen years ago, Helen came up to me and said, "Arnold, what would you think if I offered to help some of the local women who are active in the Conservative party?"

I said, "That's fine. Give them a hand if you like, but don't get *me* involved." Little did I know that years later, Helen would become president of the PC Women's Association of Nova Scotia and represent the province on the extended executive of the Conservative Women's Federation of Canada. We wound up dining or attending conferences with some of the most prominent Canadian political leaders of our time: Prime Minister John Diefenbaker, Prime Minister Brian Mulroney, Minister of External Affairs Joe Clark, Minister of Public Works Elmer MacKay, Premier Stanfield, Premier Buchanan, and Premier Bacon. And then there were Prince Edward and Princess Margaret. So Helen didn't listen to me after all!

As a kid I used to enjoy drawing in school, ever since I illustrated that poetry book in grade twelve. I carried around my crayons and pencils, and sketched outdoor scenes whenever I got a chance. As an adult I've photographed many scenes of beauty, and then gone home and painted them with oils, using the photographs as inspiration. I painted a series of seventeen oils based on photos that were taken for the royal commissions established to study the Bump. These paintings are hanging in the Miners' Museum in Springhill.

I've never sold a painting, and don't intend to: I like not being a "pro." A set of twenty-six large watercolours depicting different scenes in Springhill were exhibited at the town library for a year. Painting gives me a change of pace from emergencies.

In the fifty years that have passed since my first days as an orderly with No. 7 Canadian General Hospital, medicine has taken great leaps forward. When war broke out, sulfa, the miracle drug, was already available to cure cases of pneumonia. No longer did patients have to wait ten days to find out if they would live or die.

When I was born insulin had just been discovered. No longer did diabetics have to die after two years of misery. By the time we invaded France we were using penicillin, before the Germans had it. But it was 30,000 units dripped into the veins of the badly wounded, compared to 250,000 units in one capsule today. When I graduated from medical school we were using penicillin, streptomycin, Aureomycin, and chloromycetin. Look at the multitude of antibiotics available to doctors today.

As for diphtheria, the last time I saw it was in Belgium during the war. In 1952 and 1953, I diagnosed twenty to thirty cases of polio each year. Since the emergence of the Salk and other vaccines I have not seen another single case in my practice. Largactil came onto the market in 1953, and with its derivatives, mentally disturbed patients have been able to receive treatment that had never been available previously. Whereas before, many had been confined to institutions, today they can live useful if not absolutely normal lives in their communities. Tuberculosis sanitoriums have practically closed their doors compared to years ago, and TB patients no longer have to stay in hospital until death.

When I began my internship I saw rather quickly how many high blood pressure patients there were. At that time there wasn't much available to help them. We used phenobarb as a sedation, Apresoline, which had side effects, and veratrum veride, which was far too toxic. And finally there was the rice diet, of which I've heard more than one patient say, "I'd rather have a stroke or die than continue with that." Now we have not only multiple medications, but also surgery to increase the blood supply to the heart muscle, and in extreme cases, we can remove and replace the heart itself.

Has our quality of life changed in the past fifty years? Employment insurance, old age pensions, and Canada pensions have put more money into our pocketbooks—even when we're not working—but has all this improved our way of living? Or have some of the members of the younger generation come to believe that the world owes them a living, whether they work or not? When I grew up in the Dirty Thirties, life was so much simpler, and I was happy. Meanwhile, men have walked on the moon, computers have replaced the pen, and calculators have made math tables obsolete, but are we any happier? Sometimes I wonder about progress.

Before I went overseas nobody locked a door in Springhill, day or night. Sure, there was less to steal, but it all had greater value because people worked so hard to buy things and usually paid cash.

When I joined the army, my folks gave me a subscription to the weekly newspaper, the *Springhill Record*. Whenever I received an issue I knew everyone whose names were printed in the paper. Not only that, I knew their families, relations, and who their neighbours were. The town was always a large, close-knit family in those days.

We had a somewhat lacksadaisical attitude in school, as I recall. A phone call from the teacher to our parents would bring it to an abrupt, but temporary, halt. Today's schools have so much more to offer, yet they're appreciated even less.

Although Springhill is known for its disasters, an indomitable spirit is the town's most remarkable characteristic. People have moved away to find jobs, but many have returned to spend their retirement here. Coal has gone the way of the Edsel, but the town remains a fine place to bring up a family. The hope and true grit that motivated rescuers to risk their lives for the sake of trapped miners will live on through generations.

My fifty years of emergencies have included battle casualties, hospital care, fires, mine disasters, and more than one type of miracle. Add to this my wife and family, and this life has been well worth living. The times that I've—er, will you excuse me? The telephone's ringing....

About the Author

Dr. Robert Arnold Burden was the first doctor to go underground after an explosion rocked Springhill's No. 4 mine. Born in Springhill, Dr. Burden served in the Medical Corps from 1941 to 1945, then obtained his medical degree from Dalhousie University. After practising in Prince Edward Island, he returned to Springhill in 1957, where he was chief of staff at All Saints Hospital and served on numerous medical boards and committees.